"Straddling academia, film-criticism and polemic, this book is a wake up call to filmmakers. In applying psychoanalytic theory, the authors make a serious contribution to the literature on how to make films and their grasp of how a medium they clearly adore has been quietly hijacked by populism is truly terrifying. The films dissected here are beautifully chosen to remind us of what cinema at its best is capable of."

Andy Paterson, *Producer*, The Girl with the Pearl Earring *and* The Railway Man

"The complex failure of the American Dream is both a painful reality and, for filmmakers, an artistic opening. In this wide-ranging and sophisticated study, the authors unpack a number of key films of the Trump era, finding an astonishingly vivid portrait of the American soul in a time of cultural and moral disarray. A brilliant and challenging book that deserves a wide audience."

Jay Parini, *Novelist and Poet*, The Last Station *and* Borges and Me

"In this bold, ambitious and provocative book that will challenge and engage filmmakers, filmgoers and theorists alike, Graham S. Clarke and Ross Clarke draw on a range of theoretical approaches, including psychoanalysis, film and critical theory and social relations to produce a blistering autopsy on the American Dream through the prism of nine key films from the Trump era."

Jonathan Hourigan, *Programme Director, MA Screenwriting, University of Manchester*

"Ever since Kracauer's *From Caligari to Hitler*, film scholars have vividly described the ways in which the complex socio-political climate of an era finds indirect expression in its films. This new and compelling book by Graham and Ross Clarke casts a view beyond the usual national borders that mark such studies to provide a rich global perspective on recent cinema. Importantly, the authors show that, even as cinema changes in so many ways, this complex dynamic between films and their moment is as strong as ever."

Christian Keathley, *Professor, Film and Media Culture, Middlebury College*

"Where is the American Dream now, post Trump, in a pandemic? What is beyond the end of the end of history? This book looks at nine recent, successful and important films with a psychoanalytical analysis of character and a socio-political view on US society. A provocation, an unstable balance, that gets you thinking and arguing."

Paul Gallagher, *Head of MA Screenwriting, Birkbeck College, London University*

THE AMERICAN DREAM AND AMERICAN CINEMA IN THE AGE OF TRUMP

The American Dream and American Cinema in the Age of Trump uses both film theory and insights from object relations theory in order to examine how recent films address and reflect the state of the 'American Dream'. This fascinating book looks at how the American Dream is one of the organising ideas of American cinema, and one of the most influential cultural outputs of the twenty-first century, at a time of internal crisis.

In an era characterised by populism, climate change and economic uncertainty, the book considers nine auteur films in how they illustrate the challenges of contemporary America. Graham S. Clarke and Ross Clarke present a bifocal perspective on some of the most well-received American films of recent years and how they relate to the American Dream in the context of the Trump presidency. For each of the nine films discussed, two different accounts are presented side by side so that each film is considered from an object relations psychoanalytic point of view (internal world) as well as a film and cultural theory perspective (external world). This unique approach is complemented by discussion of political and critical theory, providing a thorough and engaging analysis.

Challenging and insightful, *The American Dream and American Cinema in the Age of Trump* will be of great interest to scholars of cinema, popular culture, American studies and psychoanalytic studies.

Graham S. Clarke is a Visiting Fellow at the Department of Psychosocial and Psychoanalytic Studies, University of Essex, UK. He has published books and papers on Ronald Fairbairn's object relations-based psychology of dynamic structure and its application to the arts.

Ross Clarke is a screenwriter and director. He is a Lecturer in Film at Met Film School, UK. His films include *Skid Row*, a documentary about the acute homeless problem in downtown Los Angeles, the dramatic features *The Birdcatcher* and *Desiree* (aka *The Chemist*) and a football documentary about Brighton and Hove Albion FC. He is currently developing a film about Jorge Luis Borges based on the book by Jay Parini.

THE PSYCHOANALYSIS AND POPULAR CULTURE SERIES

Series Editors: Caroline Bainbridge and Candida Yates
Consulting Editor: Brett Kahr

This series builds on the work done since 2009 by the Media and the Inner World research network. It aims to consider the relationship between psychoanalysis and popular culture as a lived experience that is ever more emotionalised in the contemporary age. In contrast to many scholarly applications of psychoanalysis, works in this series set out to explore the creative tensions of thinking about cultural experience and its processes whilst also paying attention to observations from both the clinical and scholarly fields. The series provides space for a dialogue between these different groups with a view to evoking new perspectives on the values and pitfalls of a psychoanalytic approach to ideas of selfhood, society, politics, and popular culture. In particular, the series strives to develop a psycho-cultural approach by foregrounding the usefulness of a post-Freudian, object relations perspective for examining the importance of emotional relationships and experience. We nevertheless welcome proposals from all fields of psychoanalytic enquiry. The series is edited by Caroline Bainbridge and Candida Yates, with Brett Kahr as the Consulting Editor.

Other titles in the Psychoanalysis and Popular Culture Series:

The Culture-Breast in Psychoanalysis: Cultural Experiences and the Clinic
by Noreen Giffney

Post-traumatic Attachments to the Eerily Moving Image: Something to Watch Over Me
by Andrew Asibong

Fantasy, Online Misogyny and the Manosphere: Male Bodies of Dis/Inhibition
by Jacob Johanssen

The American Dream and American Cinema in the Age of Trump
by Graham S. Clarke and Ross Clarke

For more information about this series, please visit: https://www.routledge.com/The-Psychoanalysis-and-Popular-Culture-Series/book-series/KARNPSYPOP

THE AMERICAN DREAM AND AMERICAN CINEMA IN THE AGE OF TRUMP

From Object Relations to Social Relations

Graham S. Clarke and Ross Clarke

Routledge
Taylor & Francis Group
LONDON AND NEW YORK

Cover image: Getty Images

First published 2023
by Routledge
4 Park Square, Milton Park, Abingdon, Oxon OX14 4RN

and by Routledge
605 Third Avenue, New York, NY 10158

Routledge is an imprint of the Taylor & Francis Group, an informa business

British Library Cataloguing-in-Publication Data
A catalogue record for this book is available from the British Library

Library of Congress Cataloging-in-Publication Data
A catalog record has been requested for this book

ISBN: 978-1-032-07268-5 (hbk)
ISBN: 978-1-032-07266-1 (pbk)
ISBN: 978-1-003-20622-4 (ebk)

DOI: 10.4324/9781003206224

Typeset in Times New Roman
by Taylor & Francis Books

CONTENTS

FIGURES

ACKNOWLEDGEMENTS

We would like to acknowledge the series editors, Caroline and Candida, for their helpful suggestions.

Graham would like to thank Sandra, for her help, forbearance and support during the development of this book and Ross for his insight and company on the journey.

Ross would like to thank Chris Keighley and Jay Parini at Middlebury College for their original impetus for this book, Nick "Lispector" Jones, Jonathan Hourigan, Andy Paterson, Nadia Conners, Teryn Fogel, Paul Gallagher, Peter Craig, Sandra Davies and Chris Briggs for the reading and comments, James Davies and all at Met Film School, Jacky, Mary, Terry and Zoe for the support, Pat's Friday Rovers, Shokoh's Curious Yellow clan, Sunday Film zoomers, Marcus and Sophie and all my students for my mental health, NWRVR and Michael Marden for sounds and most especially Dad for making a cineaste out of me.

SERIES PREFACE

The application of psychoanalytic ideas and theories to culture has a long tradition and this is especially the case with cultural artefacts that might be considered 'classical' in some way. For Sigmund Freud, the works of William Shakespeare and Johann Wolfgang von Goethe were as instrumental as those of culturally renowned poets and philosophers of classical civilisation in helping to formulate the key ideas underpinning psychoanalysis as a psychological method. In the academic fields of the humanities and social sciences, the application of psychoanalysis as a means of illuminating the complexities of identity and subjectivity is now well established. However, despite these developments, there is relatively little work that attempts to grapple with popular culture in its manifold forms, some of which, nevertheless, reveal important insights into the vicissitudes of the human condition.

The 'Psychoanalysis and Popular Culture' book series builds on the work done since 2009 by the Media and the Inner World research network, which was generously funded by the UK's Arts and Humanities Research Council. It aims to offer spaces to consider the relationship between psychoanalysis in all its forms and popular culture that is ever more emotionalised in the contemporary age.

In contrast to many scholarly applications of psychoanalysis, which often focus solely on 'textual analysis', this series sets out to explore the creative tension of thinking about cultural experience and its processes with attention to observations from the clinical and scholarly fields of observation. What can academic studies drawing on psychoanalysis learn from the clinical perspective and how might the critical insights afforded by scholarly work cast new light on clinical experience? The series provides space for a dialogue between these different groups with a view to creating fresh perspectives on the values and pitfalls of a psychoanalytic approach to ideas of selfhood, society and popular culture. In particular, the series strives to develop a psycho-cultural approach to such questions by drawing attention to the usefulness of post-Freudian and object relations perspectives for examining the importance of emotional relationships and experience.

In *The American Dream and American Cinema in the Age of Trump: From Object Relations to Social Relations*, Graham Clarke and Ross Clarke scrutinise the invitations of cinema to grapple with the political environment, offering a timely, and highly resonant, exploration of 'the American dream' and its shape-shifting meaning at a time of momentous social change. Clarke and Clarke offer a nuanced, dialogical approach – one that they describe as 'binocular', evoking a distinctive Bionian take on the work that cinema helps us to do as we work to process lived experience and attempt to *think* about its impact. The book puts the object relations psychoanalysis of Wilfrid Bion and Ronald Fairbairn into conversation with critical theory and film studies to shed light on themes encompassing prejudice in all its forms, contemporary history, emergent social movements, loss, perceptions of normality and the complex, often paradoxical, relationship between internal experience and external world events. Clarke and Clarke examine the ideological imperatives of neoliberalism by discussing nine films in the context of their production and reception, their wider social meaning and their potential for enriching the inner lives of viewers. This makes for a fascinating work, one that invites the reader into the exchange, thereby deepening our understanding of cinema as a powerful psychocultural object.

Caroline Bainbridge and Candida Yates

INTRODUCTION

The American Dream and a Binocular Approach to Analysing Film

The American Dream

In a recent essay, Churchwell (2021) has drawn attention to a common misreading of the terms of reference of the phrase 'American Dream', which she summarises in the following way, "Over time, the phrase 'American dream' has come to be associated with upward mobility and enough economic success to lead a comfortable life. Historically however, the phrase represented the idealism of the great American experiment." Churchwell points out that despite the widespread and ubiquitous misreading of the term it was always understood by the people who first popularised it as "meaning something more profound and aspirational than simple material comfort". She quotes James Truslow Adams, who in 1931 was trying to make sense of the Great Depression, which was both an economic crisis and a potential political crisis, with authoritarianism in Europe on the rise and threatening to destabilise the American political system. Adams wanted to distinguish the American Dream of a richer life spiritually, from dreams of prosperity.

> … not a dream of motor cars and high wages merely, but a dream of a social order in which each man and each woman shall be able to attain to the fullest stature of which they are innately capable, and be recognised by others for what they are, regardless of birth or position.
>
> *(Churchwell, 2021)*

In the *Epic of America* (1931) he pinpoints the frontier as one of sources of the American Dream. The idea that unlimited space led to opportunity for all, and that the frontiersman embodied a can-do spirit. A myth deconstructed in the scurrilous behaviour of the protagonists of *The Revenant* and

DOI: 10.4324/9781003206224-1

their conflicts with the Indigenous people of these new frontiers. In *Nomadland* this spirit is book-ended and examined through the lens of the working poor in America and the end of the frontier. Churchwell draws attention to a view published by the *New York Post* in 1900 warning its readers that the "greatest risk" to "every republic" was not from the so-called rabble, but "discontented millionaires" and noting that all previous republics had been "overthrown by rich men", and that this could happen in America too, where monopoly capitalists were "deriding the Constitution, unrebuked by the executive or by public opinion", and if they had their way this would be the end of the American Dream because that dream was of democracy – of equality of opportunity, of justice for all.

Churchwell notes that the other notable mention of the American Dream before Adams was by Walter Lipmann in his 1914 *Drift and Mastery*, which described what Lipmann called America's "fear economy" of unbridled capitalism. Lipmann argued that the nation's dream of endless progress would need to be restrained because it was fundamentally illusory. For Lipmann, the American Dream was the idea that the common man is inherently good and a moral barometer of the nation. Churchwell comments that "the American faith in the individual taken to its inevitable extreme creates the monstrosity of a self with no consciousness of other standards or perspective, let alone a sense of principle."

Churchwell argues that, for Adams, the American Dream was embodied in the Main Reading Room at the Library of Congress, the fundamental purpose of which was to keep democracy alive. She ventures to suggest another definition of the American Dream that needs to be revived:

> What democracy can accomplish on its own behalf for its citizens … not as a promise, or a guarantee, but as an exhortation, urging all American to do better, to be fairer, to combat bigotry and inequality, to keep striving for a republic of equals …
>
> *(Churchwell, 2021)*

The election of Donald Trump on a ticket based upon a promise of a return to the American Dream struck us as a symptom of a deep crisis in the West around the mythologies of 'the Dream'. An examination of the American Dream and its relationship to American Cinema in the era of Trump will be developed in Chapter 1 and throughout this book.

A Binocular Approach to Analysing Film

> Binocular: using both eyes to see things
>
> *(https://dictionary.cambridge.org/dictionary/english/binocular)*

This book is a binocular attempt to capture aspects of the contemporary American film industry and society as they are reflected in the films of some award winning, mostly extraterritorial, directors. We have been looking at the same films from different angles, and we value the different perspectives involved. This might usefully be compared to Bion's use of the term binocular to refer to two different perspectives: the conscious and unconscious coming together, correlating two views of the same object.

> … [Bion] writes, "The use in psycho-analysis of conscious and unconscious in viewing a psycho-analytic object is analogous to the use of the two eyes in ocular observation of an object sensible to sight" (1962, p. 86).
>
> *(Birksted-Breen, 2016)*

Or as Lene Auestad reminds us, "thinking psychoanalytically involves reflecting on how we experience everything on an unconscious as well as a conscious level, what Bion referred to as 'bifocal vision'" (Auestad, 2018). In our case, we are looking from an internal relations (unconscious) and a social relations (conscious) perspective at the meaning and implications of the films we have chosen. When Auestad comes to considering a psychoanalytic approach to prejudice, a topic taken up in Chapter 2 with Aviram's work on prejudice within a Fairbairnian outlook, she says,

> In thinking about prejudice; racism, antisemitism, xenophobia, islamophobia, sexism and homophobia I am concerned with analysing their a-rational aspect as founded in primary process logic and magical thinking, together with their social aspect as fantasies that are shared and shaped by past and present inequalities of power. Thus, psychoanalytic thinking is necessary but not in itself sufficient when it comes to grappling with these phenomena; it needs to incorporate critical reflection on its own social and cultural position. In the opposite case, what often result are analyses of the more extreme expressions of prejudice, formulated in terms of pathology, which leaves 'normality' untouched and unquestioned … Michael Balint (1969) argued that clinical experiences reveal that the structure of trauma has three phases. In the first phase the child is dependent on the adult and is in a primarily trustful relationship … In the second phase the adult, once and suddenly or repeatedly, does something highly exciting, frightening or painful. The child may be exposed to excesses of tenderness or excesses of cruelty; to severe overstimulation or rejection. The trauma is only completed in the third phase when the child, in reaction to the second phase, attempts to get some understanding, recognition and comfort and the adult behaves as if nothing had happened … In his view, the second phase is preceded by a trustful relationship, and crucially, is followed by a non-response which deprives the event of its character of reality. Bion's concept of nameless dread can be seen to point to a similar phenomenon: "If the projection is not accepted by the mother," he writes, the rejected feeling does not remain

> the same but becomes qualitatively different; it is "stripped of such meaning as it has."
>
> (*Bion, 1962, p. 116*)

Which can be seen as equivalent to what Fairbairn calls the worst thing that can happen to the developing child.

> The type of mother who is specially prone to provoke such a regression is the mother who fails to convince her child by spontaneous and genuine expressions of affection that she herself loves him as a person. Both possessive mothers and indifferent mothers fall under this category. Worst of all perhaps is the mother who conveys the impression of both possessiveness and indifference—e.g. the devoted mother who is determined at all costs not to spoil her only son. Failure on the part of the mother to convince the child that she really loves him as a person renders it difficult for him to sustain an emotional relationship with her on a personal basis; and the result is that, in order to simplify the situation, he tends regressively to restore the relationship to its earlier and simpler form and revive his relationship to his mother's breast as a partial object. A regression of this sort may be illustrated by the case of a schizophrenic youth who, whilst evincing the bitterest antagonism towards his actual mother, dreamed of lying in bed in a room from the ceiling of which there poured a stream of milk—the room in question being a room in his home just beneath his mother's bedroom. This type of regressive process may perhaps best be described as *Depersonalization of the Object*; and it is characteristically accompanied by a regression in the quality of the relationship desired. Here again the regressive movement is in the interests of a simplification of relationships; and it takes the form of a substitution of bodily for emotional contacts. It may perhaps be described as *De-emotionalization of the Object-relationship.*
>
> (*Fairbairn, 1952, pp. 13–14*)

When it comes to considering each of the films we have chosen, there will be two responses to each film. One based in Fairbairn's object relations thinking, the other based substantially in film, political and critical theory. The films weren't chosen because they exhibited the characteristics identified by some of the theories cited but because, although in the main they have been directed by outsiders to the Hollywood scene, they have been valorised both through industry-based awards and critical acclaim.

The two viewpoints that are presented in parallel are 1) an object relations view of the films we have chosen, based in the "psychology of dynamic structure" developed by Ronald Fairbairn; and 2) a view of recent contemporary culture in the US and the various conflicts that characterise the era of Trump and his "malignant narcissism". The term "malignant narcissism" was coined by psychoanalyst Erich Fromm in 1964. Later expanded by psychiatrist Otto Kernberg, who termed it a toxic combination of four highly dysfunctional traits and behaviours:

> **Narcissism,** with its grandiosity, lack of empathy, need for attention, and sense of entitlement.
> **Antisocial behavior,** with its lack of remorse, destructive and impulsive behavior, deceitfulness, and disregard for and violation of the rights of others.
> **Paranoid thinking,** with its sense of persecution, difficulty trusting others, preoccupation with others' loyalty, tendency to bear grudges, and tendency to view benign actions of others as attempts at deception or exploitation.
> **Sadism,** with its cruelty, efforts to humiliate or manipulate others, and deriving enjoyment from others' pain and suffering.
>
> *(Neurath, 2021)*

This is also the era of the hashtags Me Too and Black Lives Matter, the era of populism, the era of Covid, and the potential transformation of the culture and the economy in general, and particularly the economy and culture of the production and distribution of audiovisual content, focusing on film.

Our wider argument is that the films reflect the various failures of the 'American Dream', the attempted ideological resurrection of which, represented by 'MAGA' hats and slogans, is a crass attempt to turn the clock back to a time when America was a beacon of hope for freedom, even if this nostalgia, in itself, is problematic. This is no longer the case, as these films so effectively witness, and the slaughter, financial degradation or incarceration of the many for the advantage of the few is all too transparent.

As Candida Yates comments:

> When Trump promises to restore the nation to some notion of its former glory, he seems to offer himself up as an object of change and renewal. The performative appeal of Trump in this context can be explored through Christopher Bollas' (1987) concept of 'the transformational object'. Bollas developed Winnicott's theory of the transitional object in order to explore the world of object relating and its role in shaping subjectivity. For Bollas, the experience of transformation is linked to a dialectical movement between self and other and is bought about by the mother's adaptation to the needs of the child. Yet as a leader (and symbolic parent), Trump's version is not adaptation, but rather it is a defensive triumph over vulnerability and also the fantasies of dangerous femininity associated with the risk of the unreliable mother – as symbolised in the figure of Hilary Clinton. In this way, Trump's promise of transformation is underpinned by a wish for control – and at the level of fantasy, its collective appeal seems to operate

> culturally as a form of manic defence against the unknown and the loss of faith in the grand narrative of history and nation.
>
> *(Yates, 2018)*

A notable common feature of all the films is the trauma undergone by some or all of the principals, which makes post-traumatic stress disorder (PTSD) the most common way of understanding them.

Symptoms of complex PTSD

The symptoms of complex PTSD are similar to symptoms of PTSD, but may include:

- feelings of shame or guilt;
- difficulty controlling your emotions;
- periods of losing attention and concentration (dissociation);
- physical symptoms, such as headaches, dizziness, chest pains and stomach aches;
- cutting yourself off from friends and family;
- relationship difficulties;
- destructive or risky behaviour, such as self-harm, alcohol misuse or drug abuse;
- suicidal thoughts.

(www.nhs.uk)

Indeed, we can go further and suggest that symptoms of PTSD are what characterises the post–Second World War era as a totality. Since the early 1980s, neoliberalism has compounded these problems further. The Bomb, the Holocaust, 20 million Soviet dead, de-colonisation and neocolonialism, the continual state of war around the world, famine, mass migration, the climate crisis and the Covid pandemic ensure that none of us can sleep easily in our beds. The development since the early 1990s of Trauma Theory (www.traumatheory.com) by Alford (2018) and Radstone (2007), among others, has led to a search for, "research related to trauma theory that seeks to critique and expand the paradigm beyond psychoanalysis, beyond the West, and beyond the Holocaust of World War II" (Radstone, 2013).

There have been some notable and continuing traumas since 2000, including 9/11, the Financial Crash and attendant austerity, continuing wars in the Middle East with little improvement in the conditions or the fate of the people who are supposed to benefit, there has been runaway development of social media and surveillance capitalism and the global Covid pandemic, all of which compounds the problem of PTSD and dissociation, to say nothing of the climate crisis, with flooding, bush fires, ice caps and glaciers melting, cyclones and so on.

We have adopted the approach of presenting analysis from each perspective side by side, leaving the reader to make the connections where they can and to think about any disjunctions they notice. The reader has to actively process the arguments, finding commonality where they may and seeking agreement between the different perspectives as they might, in a parallel to the reader-response approach to film.

We hope that this will be a provocation to produce other attempts at making sense of the films discussed and of films in general, since we do not think that any one analysis or approach can exhaust the meaning of a film. Indeed, the notion of a good film, or good art, is something that is capable of promoting and sustaining a variety of interpretations.

Structure of the Book

The book is 'topped and tailed' by two short chapters, the first (this one) introducing the book and the last reflecting on aspects of the American presidential election and the defeat of Donald Trump. An approach to *Nomadland* forms an epilogue.

There are two long introductory chapters, one representing film theory and the social relations aspects of cinema in the age of Trump (Chapter 1) and the other an object relations psychoanalytic approach to the interpretation of film based in the work of Ronald Fairbairn (Chapter 2).

This is followed by nine chapters each dealing with one of the films we have chosen. Each chapter is divided into two parts – an internal world perspective, based in the object relations approach, and an external world perspective, based in film theory and social relations.

Reading Strategies

The book can be read in different ways depending upon your interests, not just from beginning to end.

If you are interested in the object relations approach to film, you can read Chapter 2 and the Internal Worlds section of each of the nine film chapters. If you are interested in the film theory and social relations aspect, you can read Chapter 1 and the External Worlds section of each of the film chapters.

If you are interested in one or a subset of the films, you can read the relevant chapter, which will include both the Internal and the External Worlds approach to each film. We believe cinema, as America's dreaming, is a way into the social and psychic life of the world.

References

Adams, J. T. (1931 / 2017) *The Epic of America*. New York: Routledge.
Alford, C. F. (2018) *Trauma, Culture and PTSD*. Palgrave Macmillan.

Auestad, L. (2018) '*Prejudice, Exclusion and the Social Unconscious*' (par EBP-BSP | Articles, Colloque du 50e Anniversaire). https://bsp-ebp.be/2018/03/31/lene-auestad-prejudice-exclusion-and-the-social-unconscious/

Bion, W. R. (1962) 'A Theory of Thinking.' In *Second Thoughts*. London: Karnac.

Birksted-Breen, D. (2016) 'Bi-Ocularity, the Functioning Mind of the Psychoanalyst'. *Int. J. Psycho-Anal.*, *97* (1): 25–40.

Churchwell, S. (2021) '*A Brief History of the American Dream*'. *The Catalyst*, 21 (Winter).

Fairbairn, W. R. D. (1952) *Psychoanalytic Studies of the Personality*. London: RKP.

Neurath, D. (2021) https://www.psychologytoday.com/us/blog/narcissism-demystified/201905/what-exactly-is-malignant-narcissism

Radstone, S. (2007) 'Trauma Theory: Contexts. Politics. Ethics'. *Paragraph*, 30 (1).

Radstone, S., Walker, J. and Shenker, N. (2013) Trauma Theory. https://www.oxfordbibliographies.com DOI: 10.1093/obo/9780199791286-0147

Yates, C. (2018) 'Reflecting on the Study of Psychoanalysis, Culture and Society: The Development of a Psycho-Cultural Approach'. *Psychoanalysis, Culture and Society*, 23 (1): 54–67.

1

EXTERNAL WORLDS

American Dream, American Nightmare: Cinema in the Age of Trump

Introduction

We began by looking for a theme or perspective that might unite the very different films that we admire, which are the subject of this book. We seized upon the idea that they each in their own way were responses to the crisis in the American Dream, the state of American democracy and the American film industry. Which, as Gramsci in the *Prison Notebooks* says of another modern 'crisis of authority', "consists precisely in the fact that the old is dying and the new cannot be born", and that it is during "this interregnum a great variety of morbid symptoms appear" (Gramsci, 1971, p. 276).

These films were developed by directors who originated, in the main, extraterritorially, and thus provide an outsider's view of the realities depicted. To us they seem, at least highly sceptical, at most deeply critical of the American Dream as anything other than an ideological caul obscuring the reality of life and its possibilities within the ambit of American life today.

While this might represent what seems to be a myopia, in that the rest of the world is ignored, it represents a deep reality in terms of the current film industry worldwide; for, even while we acknowledge the many admirable traditions and practices of film-making all around the world, they all have to survive in relation to the hegemony of American film-making and distribution. The rise of the streamers and the current trend to larger and larger acquisitions, unchecked it appears by any Anti-Trust or Monopoly laws, has seen this domination extended across the globe. This is evidenced by Amazon's 2021 acquisition of MGM for $8.7 billion, a trend successfully tested by Disney's purchase of Star Wars and Marvel Universes earlier in the century.

DOI: 10.4324/9781003206224-2

> The standardisation of world culture, with local popular or traditional forms driven out or dumbed down to make way for American television, American food, clothes, and films, has been seen by many as the very heart of globalisation.
>
> *(Jameson, 2000)*

As we began to develop our argument about the ways in which neoliberalism had hollowed out and subverted the American Dream, we were overtaken by events internationally, as the empty platitudes of neoliberalism had to face up to the realities of a worldwide pandemic and the defenders of 'there is no such thing as society' were forced to recognise our deep and continuing dependencies upon each other. We can only hope that the dramatic example of our dependency upon each other and the need for relationships within and between communities during the pandemic, will cut across the atomisation of the 'entrepreneurial self' encouraged by neoliberalism.

2020 Vision: American Dream or American Nightmare

> You hear it in every political speech, "vote for me, we'll get the dream back." They all reiterate it in similar words – you even hear it from people who are destroying the dream, whether they know it or not. But the "dream" has to be sustained, otherwise how are you going to get people in the richest, most powerful country in world history, with extraordinary advantages, to face the reality that they see around them? Inequality is really unprecedented. If you look at total inequality today, it's like the worst periods of American history. But if you refine it more closely, the inequality comes from the extreme wealth in a tiny sector of the population, a fraction of 1 percent. There were periods like the Gilded Age in the 1890s and the Roaring Twenties and so on, when a situation developed rather similar to this, but the current period is extreme. Because if you look at the wealth distribution, the inequality mostly comes from super-wealth – literally, the top one-tenth of a percent are just super-wealthy.
>
> *(Chomsky, 2017, p. 72)*

We are interested in writing about the current moment in American Cinema and the current crisis in American politics, and the ideological centre point of both is, '*The American Dream*'. Using film and social theory and object relations psychoanalysis, we will analyse popular, award winning and critically acclaimed films released during the period of Trump's campaign and Presidency and see how they reflect this 'crisis of the American Dream'. This crisis having been laid out most clearly by Noam Chomsky in his *Requiem for the American Dream* as 'The 10 Principles of Concentration of Wealth & Power' which are:

1. Reduce Democracy.
2. Shape Ideology.

3. Redesign the Economy.
4. Shift the Burden.
5. Attack Solidarity.
6. Run the Regulators.
7. Engineer Elections.
8. Keep the Rabble in Line.
9. Manufacture Consent.
10. Marginalise the Population.

Whilst acknowledging that the American Dream, "like most dreams, has large elements of myth to it. Part of the nineteenth-century dream was the Horatio Alger story, 'we're dirt-poor but we're going to work hard, and we'll find a way out,' which was true to an extent" (Chomsky, 2017, p. 64); we also recognise that the American Dream is based largely around the primacy of the individual – a particular American export of the twentieth century that has seen its natural end point in surveillance capitalism (Zuboff, 2019) and identity politics (Klein, 2020) of the last decade or more. Never has the individual been more primary, never has income disparity been so marked. Even in recession, the number of high net-worth individuals is growing at a rate of more than 30,000 per year (Neate, 2020) and the gaps between rich and poor have increased markedly since the crash of 2008 (Oxfam, 2020).

The American Dream and Cinema: Shifting Surfaces

This American Dream is perhaps best embodied in America's cinema – where most commonly a singular protagonist faces a crisis and is transformed to overcome the odds and succeed. Regardless of our feelings about the screenwriting masterclasses and somewhat overly prescriptive rule books of Syd Field (1979) and Robert McKee (1998) et al., as parodied to such great effect by Charlie Kaufman in the film *Adaptation* (2002) the transformed single protagonist, forms the basis of most American films, and more often than not the 'manna' for American Dreamers at a multiplex near you, as ubiquitous as popcorn. As Paul Schrader (2018) puts it, American Cinema is about problems, whilst European Cinema refers to dilemmas. The single protagonist of American Cinema overcomes such problems to actualise themselves – to fulfil their own individual American Dream.

Psychiatrist Vincent Deary at the beginning of his *How to Live Trilogy* recognises this model of film and how it relates to life.

> We live in small worlds. At the beginning of most movies, we are shown a status quo, more fully a status quo ante bellum, the state of things before the war. We are shown a routine and comfortable life, a small world, one that is soon to end. In screenwriting parlance, this normal, soon-to-be-over world is known as Act One, and the 'inciting incident' is the event

> that precipitates the move into Act Two, into the war of change and adjustment. And, usually, we prefer to maintain ourselves in the status quo, in comfort and predictable ease. It takes a lot to get us out of that – a compelling call, an overwhelming imperative. Or maybe we were pushed. But sometimes it happens. Things change. The moviemakers like to end Act One fairly quickly and get stuck into the spectacle of change and adjustment. That's where the drama is, that's what we pay to see.
>
> *(Deary, 2015, p. 1)*

But change is not easy and the most equitable change – social mobility – has worsened whilst the rule of law has been subverted in modern America. It is easy to see that American Cinema and the American Dream speak to and of each other. It is harder to see now, more than any other time, how the American Dream works for the many and not the few. This book sets out to see how, when real-world politics and the narrative of this Dream are in profound crisis, film speaks of this. As Winn (2007) says in his pre-recession work:

> The American Dream is a cherished belief in American Society. The United States is … the land of opportunity … Most Americans believe that this dream allows individuals to succeed without being burdened by unfair limitations. Even a poor person can through hard work and perseverance achieve success. In this way, The American Dream, is an egalitarian vision that is free of social constrains. And it is … entrenched in American popular culture.
>
> *(Winn, 2007, p. 1)*

Chomsky, amongst others (e.g., Berardi, Žižek, Zuboff) pinpoints specific ways in which the principles of social mobility and democracy are being seriously attacked and eroded in the current period. This is a moment of great change that feels unusual and groundbreaking, in the way that the late 1960s (Nixon, Vietnam, the New Hollywood) – and the late 1940s / early 1950s did (McCarthyism, the birth of TV and the end of the studio system). This moment is also a period of political and technological upheaval that influences both how films are made and distributed as well as what they might speak of. In the introduction to his study of American Cinema of the 1970s, *A Cinema of Loneliness* (2011), Robert Kolker gives historical context to the New American Cinema of that era.

> When the studios, as independent corporate bodies, fell apart in the late 1950s, assembly-line production ended. Previously each of the major studios was a self-contained filmmaking factory with its own labor pool of producers, directors, writers.
>
> *(Kolker, 2011, p. 1)*

What he goes onto describe over the opening pages not only chimes with the world of production rendered in Tarantino's *Once Upon A Time in Hollywood,* but is eerily prescient of a post Covid world where a mix of old studios and Big Tech (Warners / HBO, Disney, Amazon, Netflix, Universal / Peacock) are looking at buying up cinemas again and signing talent exclusively – effectively controlling both the means of production and the avenues of distribution – something ended suddenly by the landmark vertical integration "United States v Paramount Pictures" 1948 anti-trust case. It appears that we are returning to a new old version of the studio system, with the production chain completely integrated from production to distribution.

The 'Base' – the means of production and distribution, is changing to such a degree that we may even struggle to define what a film is – with much serialised content on TV now of cinematic quality.

The Trump Moment

The epoch herein – post-2015, is the age of Trump (wins nomination May 16, elected Nov 16), 'Me Too' (the Weinstein story breaks in *New York Times* October 2017, imprisoned February 2020), Black Lives Matter (George Zimmerman acquitted for murder of Trayvon Martin 2013, George Floyd murder and mass protests 2020), 'Time's Up' (formed January 2018) and *Netflix* (100 million subscribers July 2017; 210 million July 2021, first Emmy 2016, first Oscar 2017) – a time characterised by hugely successful populist political leaders and movements globally – epitomised by the 2016 election of Trump – scandal and resurgent identity politics in Hollywood – best characterised by the Weinstein trial and Me Too movement – and a rapidly changing technological landscape where new films, by world famous directors, can be legally downloaded and watched simultaneously on phones, tablets, TV and laptops in 192 countries thanks mainly to Netflix and now aped by a number of other Silicon Valley / Hollywood based 'streamers' in what is becoming known as "the Streaming Wars" (p. 27).

At the same time, as both authors and viewers, we have reached our own 'Hastings Limit'. The 'Hastings Limit' is a phrase coined by the editor of *The Verge,* Dieter Bohn, to describe the huge volume of content now available to stream, or to use the UK vernacular 'Box Sets'.

> I propose a new term called The Hastings Limit named after Netflix CEO Reed Hastings. He famously said that Netflix's real competition wasn't other streaming services but Sleep and Fortnite (an online gaming phenomenon) … The Hastings Limit is when you admit that there is more content than you have time for or might ever have time for.
>
> *(Bohn, 2020)*

We are restricting our remit in this book to some traditional film formats; not episodic shows – TV or streaming content, i.e., to single films between 80 and 160 minutes. We recognise that film and TV content are becoming in many cases harder and harder to distinguish. Whilst the lines are blurring daily here, with award winning series like *True Detective* and *Chernobyl* being compared to cinema in different ways, we have drawn a line to examine film or cinema as opposed to long form or episodic content.

We will examine ten films that we feel speak to the problems of the epoch in different ways, both consciously and unconsciously, and reflect a diversity of mainly external voices – particularly those we think of as 'Outsider Auteurs' e.g., non-Americans, ethnic minorities and women making American based and / or funded cinema.

The Cannes Film Festival, arguably the most important festival in existence, has epitomised the blurring of such lines and the new battlegrounds over production, form, and distribution, by simultaneously banning films produced by *Netflix* and embracing television / streaming series by their own Cannes anointed auteurs. 'Netflix Original' films were banned because they did not fulfil French law regarding the hotly contested distribution / cinema exhibition window – the long-held convention that films exhibited in cinemas would have a clear window before jumping to Airlines, SVOD, TV or DVD. Netflix has ignored this with tiny windows, or day- and date-limited releases, leading to films by auteurs like Scorsese (*The Irishman*) and Baumbach (*Marriage Story*) being excluded from Cannes. When it comes to exhibition windows and the cinemas themselves, Netflix, like other Silicon start-ups (Uber and Airbnb), has "moved fast to break things" that they see as protectionist (exhibition windows are seen as disposable as New York taxi badges and Barcelona rent housing laws). The Cannes Film Festival Director openly fell out with Netflix on this issue, as was widely reported (Wilkinson, 2018). At the same time, since 2016, Cannes has been welcoming and showcasing high-end TV / Streaming shows by preferred auteurs like Jane Campion (*Top of the Lake*) and Nic Winding Refn (*Too Old to Die Young*). Refn himself declaring his show to be "eleven hours of cinema" (as told to one of the authors by Refn himself in May 2019 at the Cannes film Festival.).

Covid has further obliterated the exhibition window as cinemas were forced to close and studios chose to transfer films to their premium streaming services (most noticeably HBO Max and Disney+). 2020 saw an acceleration of dominance for the digital platforms that might be likened to Lenin's aphorism – "There are decades where nothing happens; and there are weeks where decades happen". This is best illustrated by the growth of Disney+ predicted now to take over from Netflix as the no. 1 streamer with an audience already in excess of 100 million having only launched some 18 months ago in November 2019.

American Cinema as Dominant Cultural Export

We can agree at least that the short American Century (1941–2001/8) was a time when

> American jazz, Hollywood movies, American slang, American machines and patented products, were the only things that every community in the world, from Zanzibar to Hamburg, recognized in common.
>
> *(Rosenberg, 2012, p. 136)*

Still today, cinema box office, locally and globally, is dominated by the big Hollywood studios (Disney, Sony, Paramount, Warner Brothers, Universal and Lionsgate who have a market share of 70 per cent globally, and even more in the US) alongside the growing domination of the American owned streamers. It is easy to argue that Hollywood movies and TV (like US military forces, iPhones and pharmaceuticals) remain powerful and universally recognised even as America struggles for dominance on the world economic stage or in fact to properly provide for the needy at home. At the end of Trump's reign, regardless of debacles in Afghanistan, high COVID rates and a record homeless population at home, it remains the case that America's films and streamed content are culturally dominant in the globalised twenty-first century.

The false end of history and the real end of the dream

For a brief moment, before 9/11, the collapse of communism in 1991 seemed to usher in a dream-like decade where American capitalism had triumphed. Contrary to what Francis Fukuyama famously and fatuously described as "the end of history", the first two decades of the new century have seen changes in technology, deep economic recession, vast forced migration, an unprecedented refugee crisis and a huge shift in power eastwards. In 1992 Fukuyama said with some grandeur, no sense of hubris and to popular acclaim, that humanity has reached, "the end of history as such: That is, the endpoint of mankind's ideological evolution and the universalization of Western liberal democracy as the final form of human government" (Fukuyama, 1992). Twenty-five years later and post-Obama, Fukuyama acknowledged, in retrospect, he didn't have a sense, or a theory, about how democracies could go so far backward. Much like Chomsky's analysis, he recently wrote:

> Trump's victory also represents the latest stage in a global shift toward populist nationalism, a pattern whose meaning is starting to become frighteningly clear … That trend encompasses Brexit and the rise of right-wing anti-EU, anti-immigrant parties across Europe. In some sense, these developments – like Trump – are a delayed popular reaction to globalisation, and the economic and cultural dislocations that it has wrought in the name of a freedom that doesn't stop at the border. The "democratic" part of liberal democracy is, in other words, now rising up and taking revenge on the "liberal" part. If this trend continues elsewhere in the world we will be in for a very rough time of competing and angry nationalisms.
>
> *(Fukuyama, 2016)*

The reality of the American Dream has been in a seemingly terminal decline long before Trump. The seeds for Make America Great Again (MAGA) hats and Trump's mid-West blue-collar rebellion were laid as much by the Democrats over the preceding decades. As Emmet (2007) states:

> American culture clings doggedly to the myth of the United States as a classless society. However, in the late twentieth century, the United States led all industrial nations in income inequality ... Despite these inequalities, Americans continue to believe in the American Dream and its fundamentally promised equality.
>
> *(Emmet, 2007, p. 126)*

Worse still, the tragedy is that,

> While many Americans admit that social inequalities exist in the United States and they lead to the unfair distribution of resources, these same individuals "deemed their class inferiority as a sign of personal failure, ... even as many realised that they had been constrained by class origins that they could not control."
>
> *(Emmet, 2007, p. 127)*

For a lyrical and heart-breaking portrayal of the American Dream over the last 50 years, a reading of George Packer's *The Unwinding: Thirty Years of American Decline* (2013) is essential. A piece of nonfiction in the style of John Dos Passos's *U.S.A.* it follows a multitude of 'American Dreamers' across the decades from Reagan's 1980s to Obama's re-election and across America from Silicon Valley and Washington to inner city Ohio and broken lives in Tampa and North Carolina. Packer nails the idea of more personal freedom, at a cost, when describing what he calls "the unwinding".

> The unwinding brings freedom, more than the world has ever granted, and to more kinds of people than ever before – freedom to go away, freedom to return, freedom to change your story, get your facts, get hired, get fired, get high, marry, divorce, go broke, begin again, start a business, have it both ways, take it to the limit, walk away from the ruins, succeed beyond your dreams and boast about it, fail abjectly and try again. And with freedom the unwinding brings its illusions, for all these pursuits are as fragile as thought.
>
> *(Packer, 2013, pp. 3–4).*

He then goes on to describe how even right-wing libertarian Peter Thiel was willing to face some truths about a broken American Dream that were unpalatable to Obama's Democrats.

> On the left, there was an official smugness about innovation – just spend more money – while deep down lurked an unspoken pessimism. President Obama probably believed that there wasn't much to be done about decline except manage it, but he couldn't give another "malaise" speech (after what happened to Jimmy Carter, no one ever would again), so his picture of the future remained strangely empty. Both Obama and Romney ended up in the wrong place: the former thought American exceptionalism was no longer true and should be given up, while the latter thought it was still true. Neither was willing to tell Americans that they were no longer exceptional but should try to be again.
>
> *(ibid., pp. 385–386)*

Oprah Winfrey, poster girl of self-actualisation since the time of Fukuyama's self-proclaimed end of history, left ordinary Americans with no doubt where responsibility lay:

> Oprah's magical thinking (vaccinations cause autism; positive thoughts lead to wealth, love, and success), and watching Oprah always doing more, owning more, not all her viewers began to live their best life. They didn't have nine houses, or maybe any house; they couldn't call John Travolta their friend; the laws of the universe left them vulnerable to mugging; they were not always attuned to their divine self; they were never all that they could be. And since there was no random suffering in life, Oprah left them with no excuse.
>
> *(ibid., p. 61).*

The acknowledged long-term decline in social mobility and justice, and the unremitting ideology that, regardless of the facts, self-actualisation is available to all, led to the perfect storm of resentment that Trump's "Make America Great Again" call was welcomed by many. For the majority, locked out of wealth, the belief in real change is always fleeting and the idea of tearing the system down or even seriously reforming it merely a dream. As we shall see in our concluding chapter, Jessica Bruder's searing book *Nomadland: Surviving America in the Twenty-First Century* (2019) continues along a similar rich and tragic vein.

Some have argued that 9/11 was the death knell of the short American century, although, looking back now with further hindsight, the 2008 recession with its seismic effects on the already struggling working and underclass of America, and the launch of the iPhone that same year, were equally key events in its demise – the iPhone allowing, as it did, for the mass creation and proliferation of data harvesting, the sharing economy and social media. Essentially, *the* object of desire of the last ten years and the first hand-held portable version of what Berardi calls the *"Global Silicon Valley"* (Berardi, 2017, p. 118), the iPhone was the single most significant product of this century, in that it facilitated, through apps, what became household tech brands, and "disruptors" including **F**acebook, **A**pple, **A**mazon, **N**etflix and **G**oogle, to grow exponentially – companies known collectively by the acronym FAANG.

Certainly, this period (2001–2008), helped to create the conditions of the radical and voluntary deterioration in democracy, as described in *The Age of Surveillance Capitalism* by Shoshana Zuboff (2019) and documentaries like *The Great Hack* (2019, Jehane Noujaim and Karim Amera), as well as Netflix's exposé of Cambridge Analytica's illegal work for right-wing populists and Russian troll factories, using Facebook data. The extent of this digital threat to democracy was also unveiled repeatedly by the brave work of investigative journalist Carol Cadwalladr (2017, 2018, 2019) of the Guardian and Peter Pomerantsev in his book *This Is Not Propaganda* (2020).

As Jonathan Taplin (2017) comments on how these companies are controlling and exploiting culture:

> Modernity was constructed on the idea individuals are meant to be the ones who decide their own fates, particularly as voters and consumers. But that's not what the techno-determinist future holds. …The former editor of the Guardian Alan Rusbridger told a FT conference in 2016 that Facebook had "sucked up $27 million" of the paper's projected digital advertising revenue in the previous year. "they (Facebook) are taking all the money" he noted because "they have algorithms we don't understand, which are a filter between what we do and how people receive it". As more of our lives become digital, these new algorithmic gods will assume more power over us.
>
> *(Taplin, 2017, p. 19)*

At the same time, under a perceived ongoing crisis from 'The War on Terror' – most powerfully described in Adam Curtis's BBC documentary series – *The Power of Nightmares* (2004) we surrendered many rights long cherished by civil rights groups "in the name of "security" and then compounded the problem with the voluntary surrender of rights/data in exchange for access to social media and the internet. As the saying goes (first applied to television), "if the product is free – you are the product". For an in-depth history and critique of this maxim see Oremus (2018).

Social media and the 'War on Terror' clearly present a double challenge to freedom and democracy in the West, coupled with the systemic failures of neoliberalism to halt increasing inequality and stifle mobility and the success of so-called *Capitalism without Democracy* (Tsai, 2007) – this perfect storm leading to the rise of Trump, Bolsonaro, Brexit and worse. Peter Thiel even questioned whether Democracy and Freedom are compatible (Taplin, 2017, p. 20). At the same time, Hong Kong Umbrella movement leader Joshua Wong's story of the meeting point of Capitalism and Dictatorship as told in the Netflix documentary *Teenager vs Superpower* (2017) and his memoir *Unfree Speech: The Threat to*

Global Democracy (Wong, 2020) tells us clearly why we must act now. Hong Kong is exemplary of the problems faced by modern democracy in a globalised capitalist world. The former last outpost of the British Empire, it is now the emblematic flash point between a liberal capitalism with human rights (freedom campaigns ironically harnessed by social media) and the might of Chinese state capitalism – the modern workhouse of the world.

When thinking about privacy and data, Zuboff's major work – Surveillance Capitalism (2019) goes even further.

> Our dependency is at the heart of the commercial surveillance project, in which our felt needs for effective life vie against the inclination to resist its bold incursions. This conflict produces a psychic numbing that inures us to the realities of being tracked, parsed, mined, and modified. It disposes us to rationalize the situation in resigned cynicism, created excuses that operate like defense mechanisms ("I have nothing to hide"), or find other ways to stick our heads in the sand, choosing ignorance out of frustration and helplessness. In this way, surveillance capitalism imposes a fundamentally illegitimate choice that twenty-first century individuals should not have to make, and its normalization leaves us singing in our chains … The real psychological truth is this: *If you've got nothing to hide, you are nothing.*
>
> *(Zuboff, 2019, p. 479)*

According to Bruce Sterling, even as far back as 2011, the future came in two jokey flavours with serious undercurrents:

1. Gothic Hi-Tech: "Steve Jobs creates something brilliant, but you have to suffer from health problems."
2. Favela Chic: "You have lost everything material, no jobs or prospects, but you are wired to the gills and really big on Facebook."

The question then becomes: does capitalism need democracy and privacy to function? Successful state capitalism in China, digital monopolies, Trump's assault on the Capitol, challenges and politically motivated changes to voting rights – these all suggest democracy and capitalism may not be inevitable bedfellows. The majority of Americans now face a struggle for basic human rights in the form of access to health care, housing, education, a living wage, and real democracy whilst having access to high-speed broadband, streaming services and all the associated benefits of the internet.

The American Dream has been the single most important narrative of the short American twentieth century – most simply expressed as the idea that a peanut farmer can become president – the dream that the individual is protected by the constitution and that the class system is fluid. As outlined above it is based in ideas of democracy, social mobility and the law as enshrined in the rights of the individual in the American Constitution.

For those that still doubt the enduring power of this idea we refer you to Trump's keynote speech at Davos in January 2020, "The American Dream is back, bigger and better than ever." Donald Trump talking about what he describes as a "blue-collar boom" at Davos, of course a call back to his initial and ubiquitous election winning cry of "Make America Great Again" in 2016.

We will examine what the American Dream meant and what it now seems destined to become as Žižek's four horsemen of the Apocalypse (2010) – climate change, social disruption as evidenced by refugee crisis, biotechnology and economic disruption (to which we would add big data, surveillance and capitalism without democracy to this heady mix) challenge and dismantle it.

We will look to explore how America's foremost art form and export – cinema – has responded to the current crisis of identity. A turning inwards of America under Trump after the long-drawn-out debacle of the Iraq and Afghanistan wars, and economic emergency. A crisis of its political and social system embodied by Trump and a post-truth world dominated by social media, big tech and information harvesting. A crisis where the American Dream, as fragile as it was in the last century, has been transformed for millions in the States and around the world into what we might categorise as an American Nightmare.

Being Donald Trump: A Special Case of Crisis

> Hollywood – I don't call them the elites because I think the elites are people they go after, in many cases – but Hollywood is really terrible. You talk about racist; Hollywood is racist. What they're doing with the kind of movies they're putting out, it's actually very dangerous for our country. What Hollywood is doing is a tremendous disservice to our country.
>
> *(Donald Trump speaking to reporters,* The Guardian, *August 2019)*

The Trump presidency saw two Impeachment proceedings (one based in Russian tampering in his election as president, one a direct attack on the Capitol), his constant Twitter tirades far outside the realms of normal and long-established protocol for international diplomacy; sex scandals, most notably the Stormy Daniels affair, and the unprecedented state assassination of Qassim Suleimani. Eventually, post presidency, he was effectively banned from his own base on social media – specifically Twitter and Facebook. Trump's presidency was best categorised by the very personal nature of his attacks on those that question him and a skittish and reactionary relationship to anything approaching "objective truth". As just one example, Michael Wolff's book *Fire and Fury* (2018) about the inner sanctum of the West Wing under Trump was enough to give anyone sleepless nights about who ran the most powerful country in the world.

Trump was an outlier president, of that there is no doubt, to many a potent symbol of a world gone mad, to others, on the right, a populist prophet. As he himself said, without any irony. "And the greatest phrase, I think, in the history of politics is on all of those red and white hats that I see out there: 'Make America Great Again'" (Cilliza, 2018). The slogan is, of course, a call back itself to Ronald Reagan's 1980s poster campaign with Trump "trademarking it as early as 2012." (Martosko, 2015) No surprise here – Reagan ushered in the neoliberal dreams of Ayn Rand and Milton Friedman alongside his British counterpart Margaret Thatcher – and his relationship with cinema and Hollywood is brilliantly explored in J. Hoberman's *Make My Day: Movie Culture in the Age of Reagan* (2019).

Clearly, Trump is both a continuation of this neoliberal project, and a dangerous populist break with it. With the MAGA catchphrase and other inward looking, sometimes racist tropes, Trump has invoked a past that probably never existed, like many other populist leaders – e.g., the Colonial Empire fantasies of Farage and Johnson's Brexit or the romanticised hark backs to the Military Regime by Bolsonaro in Brazil, and by doing so he has won the support from those disenfranchised and least equipped for the ravages of twenty-first-century late capitalism or neoliberalism. This populist base perhaps best personified in all our film choices by Cleo's lover-cum-enemy Fermín in the film *Roma*.

Trump's nostalgia is for a pre-Civil Rights American utopia that never existed. The white working and lower middle class that he purports to represent are undoubtedly materially worse off in Trump's America where tax cuts have benefited only the rich and corporations. But their long-stored anger, limited by the shackles of what they see as an unnecessarily '*woke*' culture, has found its voice in Trump. Film director Todd Philips claims this very politically correct culture had prevented him making another sequel in his *Hangover* franchise and led to his turning to Joaquin Phoenix's nihilistic *Joker* to express his rage. Trump is the Joker – a fantasist and poor little rich boy who speaks for every angry white male (and some females too). He is the epitome of a world where both rich liberal movie stars and millionaire Presidents feel short changed. Everyone in Trump's America is somehow hard done by.

Everything is very personal with Trump and nothing more so than his distaste for the Democrat supporting liberal elite of Hollywood. His presidential origin story got the rocket fuel it required when he was personally roasted and ridiculed by President Obama at the White House Correspondent's Dinner in 2011. More than any other president, the worlds of entertainment and politics mix and collide in an almost surreal fashion and Hollywood plays its own part, often to its own detriment.

Quite patently the established body politic is in crisis – America itself is in crisis, probably the worst since the Vietnam War some 50 years ago. Neoliberalism has failed all but the 1 per cent – but what often emerges as 'resistance' in its place is far worse.

> The emergence of Trump in American politics, and the proliferation of nationalist regimes in the Euro-Asian continent, may be read as the formation of an anti-globalist front that unifies Donald Trump and Vladimir Putin, Jarosław Kaczyński and Viktor Orbán, Marine Le Pen and Boris Johnson. This front is the expression of the pressure of the white working class defeated by financial globalism, and it is heading for a total opposition to the neoliberal elite.
>
> *(Berardi, 2017, p. 40)*

Perhaps America has always been in crisis, the shock doctrine crisis capitalism described by Naomi Wolf (2008) has driven the economy and the military industrial complex since World War Two with wars and conflicts, internal and external from Korea to Iraq, Iran and Afghanistan, from the Civil Rights movement to LGBQT+, Black Lives Matter and Me Too. This conflict – internal and external has become, or always was the American way. The means determines the ends – America's roots as a new country formed out of European exile and mass genocide.

The Trump moment however seems to 'call back' to the schism most profoundly felt during the late 1960s and early 1970s, the struggles for racial and feminist emancipation, the protests against Nixon and Vietnam and the idea that the whole system could be torn down whilst an extreme right-wing president sits in the Oval Office. Only 50 years later, proposed alternatives and counterculture movements – not just those obsessed with single issue identity politics – seem much harder to find. The late 1960s dream of a different world has melted into air and even the railing against the 1 per cent – seen in the *Occupy Movement* for a brief moment in 2011 seems like a far-off fantasy.

> Although it seems impolite to mention it, the collapse of the "Occupy" movement over 2011–12 was largely due to the long-discredited notion that political action could be sustained and effective in the absence of any sort of theoretical guidance and hierarchical organization of short-to longer-term goals. The Tea Party had Ayn Rand; the closest thing to an Occupy inspiration seemed to be John Stewart. People seem to have forgotten that the initial Occupy Wall Street encampment on September 17, 2011, was sparked by a call from Adbusters, a "global network of culture jammers" based in Vancouver, built around a media collective and a glossy magazine. Its founder, Kalle Lasn, has asserted, "What we're trying to do is pioneer a new form of social activism using all the power of the mass media to sell ideas rather than products"
>
> *(Mirowski, 2013)*

It appears in 2021, the 1 per cent billionaires have won, and the resistance is fiercely organised solely around identity as opposed to broader class alliances – Me Too, Time's Up, Black Lives Matter. On the existential threat facing us all – the coming climate catastrophe – Americans generally take a market approach to the problem and it is Europeans like Greta Thunberg and Extinction Rebellion who call for more radical and urgent action. (See *First Reformed*, Chapter 5).

It is clear that universal rights are in retreat and yet no one seems willing or able to fight for anyone but themselves. The left is in disarray whilst all indices of inequality, poverty and income distribution are stuck hard in reverse, with epidemic homelessness the most obvious symptom in every major Western city, particularly America, and there is clear evidence that Trump's tax cuts have placed a further unnecessary burden on the poor.

In fact, bizarrely, the front-line battlegrounds of this presidency for Trump seemed to be Hollywood and the 'fake news'" media. The hope for the 2020 presidential race that Bernie Sanders and Elizabeth Warren would invoke a more radical set of ideals for Democrats than predecessors Hilary and Obama faded with the silver lining that the old guard of Biden thankfully ended Trump's reign of terror.

Warren had offered radical suggestions for what she calls the Second Gilded Age (2019) and what Berardi calls the Global Silicon Valley.

> The worldwide, scattered sphere of production in which different cultures and social interests conflict I call the Global Silicon Valley (GSV). The Global Silicon Valley has to be seen as a dynamic sphere in which conflicts are continuously emerging, as the deterritorialized sphere in which millions of semio-workers are cooperating daily for the construction of the net-automaton. We should not see this sphere only as a homogeneous field of abstract interactions. It is also a living web of connections among workers who deal with different social conditions: high-wage corporate functionaries as well as precarious designers, engineers, artists and all the inglorious workers of the net. We must look at the Global Silicon Valley, the global semio-factory, the same way Lenin regarded the Putilov plant in 1917, the same way the Italian autonomists considered the Fiat Mirafiori factory in the '70s: as the core of the production process, as the place where the maximal level of exploitation is exerted and where the highest transformative potency can be unchained.
>
> *(Beradi, 2017, p. 238)*

From a long way out, Elizabeth Warren has led American politicians' most radical and refreshing take on these Global Silicon Valley tech companies –

> It's exciting – and very hip – to talk about Uber and Lyft and Taskrabbit, but the promise and risks of these companies isn't new. For centuries, technological advances have helped create new wealth and have increased GDP. But it is policy – rules and regulations – that will determine whether workers have a meaningful opportunity to share in that new

> wealth … A century ago, the industrial revolution radically altered the American economy. Millions moved from farms to factories. These sweeping changes in our economy generated enormous wealth. They also wreaked havoc on workers and their families. Workplaces were monstrously unsafe. Wages were paltry, and hours were grueling … America's response wasn't to abandon the technological innovations and improvements of the industrial revolution. We didn't send everyone back to their farms. No. Instead, we came together, and through our government we changed public policies to adapt to a changing economy – to keep the good and get rid of much of the bad.
>
> *(Warren, 2016)*

Trump, we would agree, is right about one thing, this crisis was borne out of the intransigence or impotence of the ruling neoliberal political class to effect real change for Americans of all races, classes and sexes. More worrying still, the stuttering resistance to Trump was bogged down by a similar singular obsession with narrow identity politics as opposed to a focus on effective economic reform – here we would argue that only Sanders and Warren could have offered any hope for 'real change'.

> Darwinism is based on the idea that the fittest and the strongest will win the fight for life, and (Kevin) Kelly (*editor of Wired*) transferred this principle from the wild space of the jungle to the civilized space of the networked economy. This theory has proven right in the neoliberal age: the few individuals strong enough to exploit and plunder what is available have emerged as the winners of the late modern game. The problem is that they have almost destroyed the world. They have impoverished the working class, devastated the environment all over the planet, and pushed much of the new generation into the hell of precariousness, loneliness, and epidemic depression. At the end of the day, the neoliberal struggle for survival has generated monsters like Trump, Farage, Orbán and Duterte.
>
> *(Berardi, 2017, p. 40)*

At the same time, American Cinema's crisis chimes with the political problems of the Trump era and, as we shall see, Hollywood itself, let alone its product, is undoubtedly one of the main domestic battle grounds of his presidency, although, as we will argue, perhaps not quite in the radical ways that Trump himself suggests.

The films we have chosen were admired critically and also successful at the box office – *The Revenant, Roma, First Reformed, Sicario, Joker, You Were Never Really Here, Widows, Us, Once Upon a Time in Hollywood* and *Nomadland.* We ask if these films offer radical insights into the current moment, and the American Dream itself. Do they offer a way forward towards greater opportunities, democracy, social, racial, sexual and income equality and the rule of law or, do they at best, merely ameliorate and, at worst, reinforce the current feeling that little is possible? What do film narratives offer up not only as critique or witness to the crisis of the American Dream but as an alternative narrative or pathway for it, if any at all?

Is there a road forward for cinema? Does cinema provide a clue to movement out of this crisis? Testament to this impasse in thought in all American life is the inability to think beyond the imminent end of the world. This can most obviously be found in the moving image via the overwhelming number of zombies, apocalypse, disaster and superhero movies and TV shows churned out over the course of this new century.

Film Theory and Its Discontents: The Case for Auteurs

While the émigré / outsider director has been crucial to American Cinema throughout its history they have rarely been more successful than in the globalised twenty-first century. Me Too and Time's Up have fought for the recognition of the 'diversity' problem, rife everywhere not just in Hollywood. The outsider, as described herein, is someone defined by country of residence (outside of the USA) and / or gender and / or race. That we might take as an interesting or different perspective on America since they are not part of the dominant white male American viewpoint. In this book we will explore some recent work of seven highly successful auteurs currently working in Hollywood – two Mexican men (Cuarón and Iñárritu – *Roma* and *The Revenant*), one French-Canadian man (Villeneuve – *Sicario*), one Scottish woman (Ramsay – *You Were Never Really Here*), one Black British man (McQueen – *Widows*), one Chinese-American woman (Chloé Zhao – *Nomadland*) and an internal émigré of sorts, an African American New Yorker (Peele – *Us*). With special attention to matters of gender, race and national identity we will examine the ways in which the American Dream is refracted through their different perspectives. For contrast we will look at the recent work of three of the 'old guard' from the 1970s, the 1990s and noughties respectively – Paul Schrader's film *First Reformed*, Quentin Tarantino's *Once Upon a Time in Hollywood* and Todd Philips' comic book cross-over smash hit *Joker*.

One of the objectives is to uncover alternative ways of viewing the twenty-first-century American Dream and the tensions that exist between the rule of law and lawlessness, the law of the talion, the individual and the state, and matters of class, gender, and migration. Figures of revenge, scarcely hidden or disguised, threaten to erupt into the everyday as the possibilities of reparation are denied, the 'War on Terror' inevitably fails whilst 'the war of each against all' looms. At the end of the short American century, the American Dream, if it ever really existed, turns to a nightmare before our very eyes – one, as we have described, where law, opportunity, freedom, and security are under threat from within and without.

Each of the films chosen examines some aspect of the American Dream, including the formation of the American West and the treatment of Indigenous people, nomadic journeys across today's impoverished America, Mexico City in the late 1960s from a social realist perspective, the current criminal war on drugs on the Mexican–American border, the criminal underclass and PTSD; a female-led heist in a present-day racially divided American city and a dystopian present-future-past moment where the enemy is our doubled selves. By contrast, Schrader's film is an explicit meditation on faith and belief and what we might do in the face of the existential threat to life on Earth; Tarantino's is a barely disguised post-truth dream of a better world pre-Me Too and Netflix, whilst Philips' nihilistic comic book violence captures the zeitgeist in *Joker.*

The political and psychoanalytic aspects of these works will be read together and presented as alternative but synergetic accounts of these crucial and critically acclaimed films. The personal (internal) and the social (external) aspects of these different films will provide a way of focusing the core concerns of outsiders towards the American Dream as they are reflected in these films.

Ryan and Kellner in *Camera Politica – The Politics and Ideology of Contemporary Film* (1988) take a similar approach and offer a great introductory analysis of an earlier period (the 1980s particularly), its films and their effects, as does Kellner's 1990 follow-up *Film, Politics, and Ideology: Reflections on Hollywood Film in the Age of Reagan* (Kellner, 1990). It is no coincidence that American capitalism and cinema have a similar trajectory and timeline. They were born at similar times (the early twentieth century) and, the declaration of independence apart, the American Dream was most openly and fully enunciated in 1931 around the same time as cinema found its voice with the talkies and the advent of synced sound. Writer and historian James Truslow Adams, in his bestselling 1931 book *Epic of America*, described it as "that dream of a land in which life should be better and richer and fuller for everyone, with opportunity for each according to ability or achievement". It isn't a new idea that cinema (and TV) has long been the mouthpiece of America both at home and abroad – its not so covert ideological wing. As Kellner points out in his 1990 book:

> In our book *Camera Politica: Politics and Ideology in Contemporary Hollywood Film* (1988), Michael Ryan and I argue that Hollywood film from the 1960s to the present was closely connected with the political movements and struggles of the epoch. Our narrative maps the rise and decline of 60s radicalism; the failure of liberalism and rise of the New Right in the 1970s; and the triumph and hegemony of the Right in the 1980s. In our interpretation, many 1960s films transcoded the discourses of the anti-war, New Left student movements, as well as the feminist, black power, sexual liberationist, and countercultural movements, producing a new type of socially critical Hollywood film. Films, on this

reading, transcode, that is to say, translate, representations, discourses, and myths of everyday life into specifically cinematic terms, as when *Easy Rider* translates and organizes the images, practices, and discourses of the 1960s counterculture into a cinematic text. Popular films intervene in the political struggles of the day, as when 1960s films advanced the agenda of the New Left and the counterculture. Films of the "New Hollywood," however, such as *Bonnie and Clyde, Medium Cool, Easy Rider*, etc., were contested by a resurgence of right-wing films during the same era (e.g. *Dirty Harry, The French Connection*, and any number of John Wayne films), leading us to conclude that Hollywood film, like U.S. society, should be seen as a contested terrain and that films can be interpreted as a struggle of representation over how to construct a social world and everyday life.

(Kellner, 1990)

Netflix and the Big Four: Delivering a Streaming Kind of Crisis?

> Technologies that change society are technologies that change interactions between people.
>
> *(Hidalgo, 2015)*

'The streaming wars' have been used to describe the upsurge in competition for digital content streaming services both in America and globally. Streaming services differ from traditional cable or terrestrial TV in that they are "streamed" over internet cloud services (dominated by Amazon as the number one cloud provider) to individuals, they aren't restricted by schedule (e.g., all programming is released and available to watch 24/7 without adverts) and often 'stream' in multiple territories and can be watched across these by all users.

In an ironic twist, given his key role as the second most famous cancellation in the Me Too revelations, the actor Kevin Spacey; the man that built Netflix with his game-changing show *House of Cards* – in a Mactaggart lecture in Edinburgh in 2013 talked about the third Golden Age of Television Spacey (2013) and offered a fairly prescient prediction about the successes of the 'streamers' to come:

> We have learned the lesson that the music industry didn't learn, give people what they want, when they want it, in the form they want it in, at a reasonable price, and they'll more likely pay for it rather than steal it. Well, some will still steal it, but I believe this new model can take a bite out of piracy.

Despite this self-declared third Golden Age of Television, there is a paucity of literature on the explosion of content, and a guide to TV and streaming from an academic perspective is urgently needed. This is not that book, but we acknowledge the influence and impact of these changes on film-making, film-makers and the future of cinema. The pandemic and streaming have led to a huge increase in production of TV or episodic content and a definite crisis in cinema and film production, the outcome of which is still unclear for cinema. Independent cinema has always managed to reinvent itself, but which feat of escapology it pulls in this accelerated epoch of digital dominance in distribution is unclear.

Historical Conditions of the Crisis: What Is to Be Done When There Is Nothing to Be Done?

> History is not like some individual person, which uses men to achieve its ends. History is nothing but the actions of men in pursuit of their ends.
>
> *(Karl Marx and Friedrich Engels,* The Holy Family, *1844)*

When we ask what is to be done, as Schrader does in *First Reformed*, we are reminded of a recent Philip Pullman article about the "disgrace of homelessness".

> We need individual acts … of course. But they're just drops of water when what we need is a flood. We need political change – by all means. Let's have a system that liberates us instead of choking the possibility of a decent life for everyone. But I'm coming more and more to believe there's something in us that relishes wickedness and nourishes stupidity, something much deeper than political systems or economic theory … Nothing can grow in this poisoned wilderness except money. Shame, which needs the soil of conscience before it can take root, can't flourish here; little shoots tentatively appear, only to fade and droop and die in the corrupted air. Imagine Boris Johnson expressing shame. Imagine Donald Trump doing so. Why feel shame? Who needs shame? Shame is for losers.
>
> *(Pullman, 2019)*

This all-important question "What is to be done?", an echo of Lenin's 1902 call, is unanswered by the left, whilst it is left to children to call for real radicalism. As embodied by climate change activist Greta Thunberg in her most famous speech:

> We must change almost everything in our current societies.
> The bigger your carbon footprint – the bigger your moral duty.
> The bigger your platform – the bigger your responsibility.
> Adults keep saying: "We owe it to the young people to given them hope."
> But I don't want your hope.
> I don't want you to be hopeful.

> I want you to panic.
> I want you to feel the fear I feel every day.
> And then I want you to act.
> I want you to act as you would in a crisis.
> I want you to act as if our house is on fire.
> Because it is.
>
> *(Thunberg, 2019)*

And at the same time, Žižek talks about this problem of "action" or what action to take.

> There should no longer be any doubt: global capitalism is fast approaching its terminal crisis. We have identified the four horsemen of this coming apocalypse: the worldwide ecological crisis; imbalances within the economic system; the biogenetic revolution; and exploding social divisions and ruptures. But if the end of capitalism seems to many like the end of the world, how is it possible for Western society to face up to the end times?
>
> *(Žižek, 2010)*

In a major analysis of our global situation, Žižek argues that our collective responses to economic Armageddon correspond to the stages of grief: ideological denial, explosions of anger and attempts at bargaining, followed by depression and withdrawal (op. cit. Introduction).

> What, then, is to be done? How are we to choose between the three main options: (1) the "Bartleby politics" of doing nothing; (2) preparing for a radical violent act, a total revolutionary upheaval; (3) engaging in local pragmatic interventions? …… Today, we do not know what we have to do, but we have to act now, because the consequences of inaction could be catastrophic.
>
> *(op. cit.)*

The accelerated changes of the early twenty-first century – the rise of China, 9/11, the crash of 2008, the dominance of tech and FAANG, the sharp acceleration of climate change, the ongoing populist wave and now a global pandemic have seen Capitalism surviving in ways that couldn't be predicted. 'Capitalism without Democracy' is a particularly dramatic and, increasingly popular, idea and practice. But Zuboff's Orwellian *Surveillance Capitalism* (2019) offers a sobering corrective to Thomas Piketty's overly optimistic *Capital in the Twenty-First Century* written just seven years ago. Post Brexit, Bolsonaro and Trump, Piketty's book already feels from another more hopeful, even naïve, time. Although Piketty's comments on the United States seem in line with Chomsky's comments,

> … on the one hand this is a country of egalitarian promise, a land of opportunity for millions of immigrants of modest background; on the other hand, it is a land of extremely brutal inequality, especially in relation to race.
>
> *(Piketty, 2013)*

Impotence to change this descent, this race to the bottom, to an end of democracy and even global extinction seems to be the accepted wisdom of the left. At the time of writing, the impact of Biden is hard to gauge, domestically his efforts feel like the boy who put his finger in the dike – it will clearly take more than one president to reverse the tide of 40 years of history.

We acknowledge that in order to analyse the present we must consider the past as well as possible futures – and we are attempting to take the period of the Trump presidency as a snapshot of the ongoing moment. This is a time of undoubted Western crisis when the future seems exclusively apocalyptic – the oft used slogan of the left – "the end of the world was / is easier to imagine than the end of Capitalism" has been repeated so often it has lost all its power or urgency and Žižek's idea that we are "Living in the End Times" seems almost trite, an empty truism. Cinema in the last decade has provided us with numerous almost infinite such end points – apocalyptic and post-apocalyptic – the Anthropocene writ large on screen. We write this as a global pandemic (COVID-19) looms large, adding further to the sense of apocalyptic times. In one year, we've gone from a world where the new James Bond film has just been pushed from April 2020 to September 2021 release, festivals are now often virtual, and HBO and Warner's have moved their entire cinematic offering online in the US for 2020/21. Cinema, like America, is in crisis – as ever it is not outside the world, and it speaks to the world.

Perhaps the current moment is best illustrated by IMDB's most popularly rated TV show ever, the mini-series *Chernobyl*. Historically the Chernobyl incident was of course part of the death knell of the Soviet Union, a symbolic precursor of the collapse of the system. In the mini-series, a man fights to save the world. He succeeds by sacrificing the lives of many working-class people and by playing along with the lies of the state in a pragmatic fashion for the greater good. It is a noble and necessary lie, but once the Chernobyl crisis is averted, he then realises it is probably not a world he wants to live in anymore. He has saved a world where corruption is bleak and omnipresent, its lies so opaque, and the opportunity for change is so meagre that the story is book ended with his own suicide. The show, part history, part Kafkaesque / hyper-normalised world stands in as allegory for our current moment. A moment where the act of a noble individual will NOT change the system it saves from itself and lies are commonplace. In 2020, Soviet state communism stands in for the current moment. Lies, hopelessness, power, and profit always before people.

As Chernobyl ushered in the end of communism, we might consider the end of this opposition to the West, "Communism didn't topple capitalism but kept it honest – and so saved it from itself" (Chakrabatty, 2019).

Adam Curtis's series *Can't Get You Out of My Head* talks about the recent failure of the left to change the world. Is cinema just a witness to this? As he says,

> When you had the rise of Thatcher and Reagan in the 1980s, the Left and liberals retreated into culture, thinking they could change things from there. But things didn't change. I believe the role of art is to express its time beautifully. And in a funny way, how it's doing that now is by beautifully expressing the paralysis of our age. Culture is a comfort blanket that radicals cling to so they can hide from the terrible fact that they don't have any answers.
>
> *(Curtis, 2021)*

The Trump presidency is over, but America is as divided as it has ever been around identity – race, diversity, gender, sexuality. The age of the individual has led America to look even further back into its violent past. At the same time the future – Big Tech – and its ascendancy has been firmly established by the COVID crisis. Looking back, the last five years seems like an eternity. We hope analysing these films provides some sense of the way we were. Some sense of the way we might be.

Cinema is, without doubt, on the brink of radical change, with the streamers now becoming 'the new studios' in both production and distribution. These films represent the last American Cinema of an age before the streamers achieved complete dominance.

Out there on the streets of America, no one can ignore the scenes of violent conflict and police shootings from the summer of 2020, the storming of the Capitol in January 2021, the death of more than 972,000 (and rising) from COVID-19 – these are the signs and symbols of the current American Nightmare.

References

Agree Staff (2013) 'Reagan's 1980s poster campaign'. http://www.iagreetosee.com/portfolio/make-america-great-again/ (last accessed Mar 2020).

Bastani, A. (2019) *Fully Automated Luxury Capitalism*. London: Verso.

Beradi, F. (2015) *Heroes: Mass Murder and Suicide*. London: Verso.

Beradi, F. (2017) *Futurability: The Age of Impotence and the Horizon of Possibility*. London: Verso.

Bohn, D. (2020) '*Hastings Limit*'. https://www.theverge.com/2020/1/17/21069703/streaming-wars-peacock-subscription-fatigue-exhaustion-apple-hbo-hulu-netflix-quibi-disney-augh (last accessed Mar 2020).

Cadwalladr, C. (2017) 'The great British Brexit robbery: how our democracy was hijacked'. *The Guardian, 7 May*. ISSN 0261–3077.

Cadwalladr, C. and Graham-Harrison, E. (2018). 'Revealed: 50 million Facebook profiles harvested for Cambridge Analytica in major data breach'. *The Guardian*, March. ISSN 0261–3077.
Cadwalladr, C. (2019) 'The Great Hack: the film that goes behind the scenes of the Facebook data scandal'. *The Observer*, 20 July 2019. ISSN 0029–7712.
Chakrabatty, A. (2019) 'The task of politics today…'. *The Guardian*, 14 Nov.
Chomsky, N. (2017) *Requiem for the American Dream: The 10 Principles of Concentration of Wealth & Power*. Seven Stories Press.
Cilliza, C. (2018) https://edition.cnn.com/2018/06/21/politics/donald-trump-minnesota-speech/index.html (last accessed Mar 2020).
Curtis, A. (2021) *Can't Get You Out of My Head.*
Deary, V. (2015) *How We Are (How to Live Trilogy* Vol. 1). London: Penguin Books.
Ellwood, G. (2019) *Too Old to Die Young*. https://collider.com/too-old-to-die-young-review-nicolas-winding-refn/9 (last accessed Mar 2020).
Emmett Winn, J. (2007) *The American Dream and Contemporary American Cinema*. Bloomsbury Academic: London.
Field, S. (1979) *Screenplay – The Foundations of Screenwriting*. Delta Books.
Fukuyama, F. (1992) *The End of History and the Last Man*. Free Press.
Fukuyama, F. (2016) 'America – the failed state'. *Prospect Magazine*, Dec.
Gramsci, A. (1971) *Selections from the Prison Notebooks*, eds. G. Hoare, and G. Nowell Smith. New York: International Publishers.
Hidalgo, C. (2015) *Why Information Grows: The Evolution of Order, from Atoms to Economies*. London: Allen Lane.
Hilmes, M. (2003) *The Television History Book: Television, Media & Cultural Studies*. London: BFI.
Jameson, F. (2000) 'Globalization and Political Strategy'. *New Left Review*, July/Aug.
Klein, E. (2020) *Why We're Polarized*. London: Profile Books.
Kellner, D. (1990) *Film, Politics, and Ideology: Reflections on Hollywood Film in the Age of Reagan*. UCLA Press.
Kolker, R. (2011) *A Cinema of Loneliness*, 4th Edition. Oxford University Press.
Lyons, K. (2019) 'Alec Baldwin tweets back as Donald Trump talks of "retribution" for SNL'. *The Guardian*. https://www.theguardian.com/us-news/2019/feb/18/donald-trump-talks-of-retribution-after-alec-baldwin-parody-on-snl (last accessed Mar 2020).
Martosko, D. (2015) '*Trump trademarked slogan'. Daily Mail*. http://www.dailymail.co.uk/news/article-3077773/Trump-trademarked-slogan-Make-America-Great-just-DAYS-2012-election-says-Ted-Cruz-agreed-not-use-Scott-Walker-booms-TWICE-speech.html (last accessed Mar 2020).
McKee, R. (1998) *Story – Style, Structure, Substance, and the Principles of Screenwriting*. London: Harper Collins.
Mirowski, P. (2013) *Never Let a Serious Crisis Go to Waste*. London: Verso.
Neate, R. (2020) 'The super-rich'. *The Guardian*, https://www.theguardian.com/news/2020/mar/04/the-super-rich-another-31000-people-join-the-ultra-wealthy-elite (last accessed Mar 2020).
Niemi, R. (2016) *The Cinema of Robert Altman (Directors' Cuts)*. Columbia University Press.
Oremus, W. (2018) 'Are you really the product?' *Slate* https://slate.com/technology/2018/04/are-you-really-facebooks-product-the-history-of-a-dangerous-idea.html (last accessed March 2020).

Oxfam (2020) 'Five shocking facts about extreme global inequality'. https://www.oxfam.org/en/5-shocking-facts-about-extreme-global-inequality-and-how-even-it (last accessed Mar 2022).

Packer, G. (2013) *The Unwinding: Thirty Years of American Decline.* Faber and Faber.

Piketty, T. (2013) *Capital in the Twenty-First Century.* London: Harvard University Press.

Pullman, P. (2019) '*Homelessness is a national disgrace*'. *The Guardian*, Dec 2019.

Rosenberg, E. S. (2012) 'Consuming the American Century'. In Andrew J.Bacevich *(ed.) The Short American Century.* Harvard University Press.

Ryan, M. and Kellner, D. (1988) *Camera Politica – The Politics and Ideology of Contemporary Film.* Indiana University Press.

Schrader, P. (2018) *Paul Schrader looks back.* https://www.newcityfilm.com/2018/05/22/flashback-first-reformeds-paul-schrader-looks-back-back-in-mid-career/. Chicago: New City Film.

Spacey, K. (2013) 'Kevin Spacey: television has entered a new golden age '. *The Guardian.* https://www.theguardian.com/media/2013/aug/22/kevin-spacey-tv-golden-age (last accessed Mar 2020).

Sterling, B. (2011) https://bigthink.com/endless-innovation/bruce-sterlings-scenarios-for-the-future-favela-chic-and-gothic-hi-tech (last accessed Mar 2020)

Taplin, J. (2017) *Move Fast and Break Things: How Facebook, Google, and Amazon Have Cornered Culture and What It Means for All of Us.* London: Macmillan.

Thunberg, G. (2019) *No One Is Too Small to Make a Difference.* London: Penguin.

Tsai, K. S. (2007) *Capitalism without Democracy: The Private Sector in Contemporary China.* Cornell University Press.

Warren, E. (2016) 'Remarks by Senator Elizabeth Warren "Strengthening the Basic Bargain for Workers in the Modern Economy"', New America Annual Conference. https://www.warren.senate.gov/files/documents/2016-5-19_Warren_New_America_Remarks.pdf (last accessed Mar 2020).

Wilkinson, A. (2018) "Netflix vs Cannes". *Vox.* https://www.vox.com/culture/2018/4/13/17229476/netflix-versus-cannes-ted-sarandos-thierry-fremaux-okja-meyer owitz-orson-welles-streaming-theater (last accessed Mar 2020).

Williams, R. (1974) *Television: Technology and Cultural Form.* Routledge Classics.

Wolf, N. (2008) *The Shock Doctrine: The Rise of Disaster Capitalism.* London: Penguin Books.

Wolff, M. (2018) *Fire and Fury.* Little Brown.

Wong, J. (2020) *Unfree speech: The Threat to Global Democracy and Why We Must Act, Now.* Penguin Books.

Žižek, S. (2010) *Living the End Times.* London: Verso.

Zuboff, S. (2019) *The Age of Surveillance Capitalism.* Profile Books Ltd.

2

INTERNAL WORLDS

Fairbairn's Psychology of Dynamic Structure

Object Relations, Psychoanalysis and Neoliberalism

Over the past few years there has been increasing interest and research into the effect of neoliberalism on the development of persons. Neoliberalism has often taken the form of an attack on our needs to relate to and depend upon others and our need for others in order to flourish. This is by no means unequivocal, but we think that those thinkers who are influenced by object relations psychoanalysis are correct when they argue that human beings are intrinsically social and relational and that to deny either of these aspects is to potentially damage a person's ability to flourish. We think that those thinkers who have identified neoliberalism as an attack on dependency and interdependency, for instance Layton (2013) and Rustin (2013), are right. We aren't naturally atomic individuals that pursue selfish goals as rational agents, we are naturally emotional and rational agents that pursue social goals within and for our communities. In terms of our understanding of real interdependence, this is not a form of identification but the ability to work with properly differentiated others. Insofar as the social order encourages denial of basic human needs, leading to splitting and fragmentation, it encourages the development of schizoid individuals. We think that Fairbairn's psychology of dynamic structure is based upon the essentially social and relational needs shared by everyone, and later in this chapter we will suggest how his thinking might be applied to an understanding of films.

Over the past decade or so, since the economic crash of 2007–2008 and the years of austerity imposed on ordinary people while bankers and others responsible for the financial crisis escaped more or less scot-free, there have been a number of attempts to understand the consequences of neoliberalism both socially and psychologically. We will consider a few of these to try and locate the continuing crisis to which the films we have chosen are responding.

DOI: 10.4324/9781003206224-3

> [T]he financial crisis has been used by many Western governments as a means of further entrenching the neoliberal model. They have adopted swingeing 'austerity measures' which, they claim, is the only way of reducing the deficits generated during the bonanza period of the 1980s and 1990s. They have launched an assault on the incomes, living standards and conditions of life of the less well-off members of society. In the UK, the cuts programme has frozen incomes, capped benefits, savaged public sector employment and undermined local government. It has encouraged private capital to hollow-out the welfare state and dismantle the structures of health, welfare and education services. The burden of 'solving' the crisis has been disproportionately off-loaded on to working people, targeting vulnerable, marginalised groups. These include low-income, single parent families; children in poverty; women juggling part-time employment with multiple domestic responsibilities; pensioners, the disabled and the mentally ill; welfare-benefits and low-cost public housing 'dependents'; the young unemployed (especially black youth); and students. Youth facilities have been closed; and citizens who depend on public amenities for their social well-being find themselves bereft.
>
> *(Rustin, 2013, p. 4)*

A significant aspect of this and other psychoanalytically informed responses is prompted by Foucault's assertion that we have all become entrepreneurs of our own lives now under neoliberalism.

> Foucault (2008: 226) has argued, 'the stake in all neoliberal analyses is the replacement every time of homo oeconomicus as partner of exchange with a homo oeconomicus as entrepreneur of himself'. Under neoliberalism, the enterprise form is extended 'to all forms of conduct' … and encompasses subjectivity itself … In contrast to classical liberalism, neoliberalism does not assume that conduct automatically takes on an entrepreneurial form; instead, neoliberal regimes develop institutional practices for enacting this vision.
>
> *(Scharff, 2016)*

Peter Gillespie (2018) has offered a Lacanian account of neoliberalism beginning in 1938 at the Walter Lippmann Colloquium,

> This forum brought together corporate, state, and academic actors for the purpose of revitalizing 19th-century liberalism in the wake of the Great Depression and the subsequent "crisis of capitalism."

Which led on to the Mont Perelin Society conference in 1947 organised by Friedrich Hayek and the formalisation of neoliberal principles.

> The first of the core principles of neoliberalism is that the market is the sovereign information processing system – more effective than any individual, group, or government…

This led in 1949 to Ludwig Von Mies concluding that

> From the neoliberal perspective it doesn't matter whether an action stems from clear rational deliberation or is the result of forgotten memories and repressed desires, because the important point is that *an action has been taken*. With this comparison, neoliberalism attempts both to incorporate and displace, if not marginalize, the importance of psychoanalysis to political theory and practice … The third fundamental concept of neoliberal thought concerns a new theory of the subject. Neoliberalism completely abandons the classical liberal conception of 'economic man.' In classical liberalism economic man is viewed as a rational and autonomous individual entering the marketplace with all the necessary knowledge to make appropriate and rational choices based on his or her own unique desires and needs. This conception is replaced in neoliberalism with a new political subject that is irrevocably divided between knowledge and ignorance, thought and action, and risk and uncertainty.

And

> The final element of neoliberalism is the concept of "the entrepreneur of the self" introduced by Foucault in his 1978–1979 lectures … The goal is ultimately to shape and guide people's thoughts, affects, and behaviors through market mechanisms … the "free" market is the sovereign information processing system … located in the position of truth. In these terms, neoliberalism should not be seen as resulting from the cynical manipulation of existing democratic processes for the benefit of a global elite but as a regime of truth, the unconscious truth of the contemporary social link.

Ending with what he calls the underlying truth of neoliberalism, an echo of Foucault's point, "namely that *people have become corporations*, where the success or failure of any human encounter is evaluated in terms of the return on one's investment" (Gillespie 2018). There have been a number of attempts by psychoanalytically informed commentators to understand the psychic changes that the dominant neoliberal ideology and practice engenders and enforces. Whilst our book is not aimed at developing this body of theory, it does live within the horizon of such thinking, and we expect that, when analysed using Fairbairn's theory, the films will display several of the psychic distortions highlighted by these theorists of neoliberalism's effects on psyche and society (Layton 2013, 2014a, 2014b; Rustin 2013). In the abstract to her 2012 paper on 'Historicising Subjectivity' Layton says:

> My purpose is to ground psychoanalytic theory about what humans need in history and so to question what it means to talk ahistorically about what humans need in order to thrive psychologically. Only in so doing can one assess the relation between psychoanalysis and progressive politics. I conclude that while psychoanalysis is a discourse of its time, it can also function as a counter-discourse and can help us understand the effects on subjectivity of a more than thirty-year history in the West of repudiating dependency needs and denying interdependence.

In 2014, Layton made her critique more explicit in discussing 'Some psychic effects of neoliberalism: Narcissism, disavowal and perversion' from an object relations perspective when she writes:

> Neoliberalisms promote the development of certain versions of subjectivity, certain character structures, defenses, transferences, and countertransferences. Foucauldian theories go only so far in being able to account for the way neoliberal versions of subjectivity are lived. The paper elaborates on the individual, group, and relational effects of social repudiations of vulnerability and dependency needs and describes the perverse effects of the widespread disavowal of the interdependence of privileged and marginalized populations.
>
> *(Layton, 2014a, p. 161)*

Where,

> My conception of narcissistic process and character derives from a mix of psychoanalytic theories of narcissism, dissociation, disavowal, and schizoid phenomena; predominant influences are Kohut (1971, 1977), Klein (1946), Sullivan (1953), Fairbairn (1954), and Guntrip (1971).
>
> *(Layton, 2014a, p. 165)*

In another paper of the same year on 'Grandiosity, Neoliberalism and Neoconservatism' she argues that

> grandiosity, on both the individual and the collective level, is in part a response to dramatic cultural changes, particularly the solidification of neoliberalism in the '80s and '90s, which led to vast inequalities in income and to the increasing privatization of formerly public goods and services. Along with the income inequalities that have produced a lot of parental anxiety about their and their children's class status, neoliberal practices have encouraged a denial of dependence and interdependence. This, in turn, has produced fragile self-states marked by, for example, oscillations between grandiosity and self-deprecation.
>
> *(Layton, 2014b, p. 463)*

Rustin, in his contribution to the possibility of a relational society in the *Kilburn Manifesto* (1915), talks about the fundamental needs of human beings, their development and an appropriate social milieu for them to flourish within, in terms that echo those used by Fairbairn in the 1940s when he developed his psychology of dynamic structure.

> Our argument is that the entire basis of this debate – the idea of the autonomous, self-seeking individual as the foundational 'atom' of the human world – is wrongly conceived. For human beings are essentially social beings – and individual freedom and choice, where they emerge and exist, are the outcome of delicate and precarious social arrangements, not primordial facts of nature.
>
> *(p. 2)*

> Human beings come into the world entirely helpless, and are dependent, for many years, on the care of others. Indeed, they are even dependent, as human scientists now tell us, on their loving care, since the capacity of persons to develop minds and emotional resources depends on the quality of attention given to them through their infancy and childhood. Throughout their lives, but in particular in their later years, people are vulnerable to illness, and nearly all will experience a period of time when they are as intensely vulnerable and dependent upon the ministrations of others as they were when they were first born
>
> *(p. 3)*

> The development of human potentialities and capabilities, and thus the potential both for individuals' fulfilment and for the production of social goods, depends essentially on the quality of relationships within which they are nurtured. This is a proposition to which we think a redesign of our economy and social system needs to give deep attention.
>
> *(p. 11)*

As we develop the Fairbairnian approach we have adopted, you should be able to see the deep similarities between this fundamentally relational approach and the one we have adapted for the analysis of films and dreams.

Alternatives to Neoliberalism

One of the main factors in the multiple crises we have identified, which we argue are the subject of the films we will analyse, is neoliberalism. It is fitting therefore to initiate, at some level, a brief search for coherent alternatives to neoliberalism that might be capable of allowing us not just to imagine a future in which we and the earth might flourish but to also find ways of working practically to realise that. We have already mentioned some of the approaches to understanding, criticising and moving beyond neoliberalism in the work of the various oppositional movement to big business, big pharma and ecological catastrophe. One such initiative in the UK is the *Kilburn Manifesto* (Hall et al., 2015) but there are many others.

In what may turn out to be a very prescient move, Slavoj Žižek has edited and helped publish Frederic Jameson's *An American Utopia: Dual Power and the Universal Army* (Verso, 2016). This book contains Jameson's original essay and a number of responses to it "Although the reactions are often critical towards Jameson, they all agree on the need to radically rethink the leftist project" (Žižek, p. vii). One approach to finding an alternative to the cul-de-sac of neoliberalism is the debate that has been started around *An American Utopia.* Jameson mourns the recent dearth of new utopian thinking, the origins of which he places at around the time that Ernst Callenbach's 1975 book *Ecotopia* was published. He suggests that it was,

> the triumph of Reagan-Thatcher deregulation in the late 1970s and early 1980s that spelled the end of utopian thinking, at the same time that it seemed to seal the victory of late capitalism over all imaginable, let alone practicable, alternatives.
>
> *(Jameson, 2016, p. 1)*

In a discussion of *An American Utopia* (March 2014) at CUNY between Jameson and Stanley Aronowitz, Jameson says "This kind of transformation, this utopian army … only happens in emergencies…it is only in a national emergency … and those things are probably coming". He was, he says later, thinking of the climate crisis as the precipitating event of such a move but the current coronavirus pandemic, which may also be deeply related to the climate crisis, has led to the sort of emergency when innovative and utopian thinking of this sort is required and might be crucially necessary for us to make the sorts of adjustment to the new reality that will be needed. There is a sense in which these films and their meanings are the equivalent of the canary in the coal mine alerting us to otherwise invisible toxins we would do well to avoid. These toxins will concern ways of relating, or failing to relate, to our fellows, and failures of appropriate empathy and dependency towards workers in the NHS, for instance, whose reality is denied by the panic-buying hoarders, and other obvious pathologies of the body politic, that we avoid or ignore at our peril. It is here that the 'constructions of subjectivity' will have to be worked over practically and challenged in the everyday world of individual personal and social experience.

What these films show is the daily struggle to resist the pressures to split, to fraction, to atomise, and to treat oneself as a flexible, entrepreneurial, 'all things to all men' bundle of conditioned responses, until all that is left are uncoordinated ego-nuclei (Glover 1932), functionaries, lickspittles. Where the form of the film is more like an allegory, or an origin story, we are faced with irreconcilable difference, the fight of each against all, or as Hobbes put it, “Bellum omnium contra omnes”, not as a state of nature at all but the consequences of the ‘civilising’ power of the neoliberal state.

Fairbairn: Endopsychic Structure, the Interpretation of Dreams and the Interpretation of Film

Introduction

In the second edition of his book Sex, *Death and the Superego*, Ronald Britton (2021), a doyen of the British Psychoanalytic Society, offers the following re-assessment of the work of Ronald Fairbairn.

> When I began reviewing my ideas on the need to reconstruct the underlying metapsychological assumptions of psychoanalysis, I thought of myself as taking a new path, but I soon found out that I was stepping into the footsteps of an earlier pioneer, Ronald Fairbairn.
>
> *(Britton, 2021, p. 2)*

Britton goes on to note the generally unrecognised importance of Fairbairn’s work and in particular his contribution to the ‘Controversial Discussions’ (King and Steiner, 1991, pp. 358–361).

> It was concise, clear and enormously relevant to the discussions. It was ignored completely, and his opinions subsequently were not taken up … the neglect of his critique and subsequent modification of Freud’s structural model may have more to do with his being in Edinburgh, far from London, than their content.
>
> *(Britton, 2021, p. 3)*

As Britton commented in a recent Webinar (28 Nov 2020), under the auspices of the Melanie Klein Trust, talking to David Tuckett about updating his book originally entitled *Sex, Death and the Superego* (2003).

> My new ideas were anticipated years ago by Ronald Fairbairn, which I reread, hadn’t read that for years. Very much neglected in London … At the height of the controversies, so-called … about Melanie Klein’s ideas … Fairbairn who worked and lived in Edinburgh sent a very cogent short piece (King and Steiner, pp. 358–61) which if they had paid attention to it would have spared them a lot of trouble in the discussions … those ideas … were completely disregarded as if he had never contributed at all …

There is also explicit testimony to the importance of Fairbairn’s work from the website of the Institute of Psychoanalysis.

> One of Fairbairn's major theoretical developments was his delineation of a psychological model of the mind, departing from Freud's biological theory ... Fairbairn asserted ... that what is primary in us all is our search for relationships, and that this is more urgent than the desire to gratify instincts ... Fairbairn's emphasis on the centrality of relationships in the psyche was a great inspiration to John Bowlby and played a key role in the development of Bowlby's famous 'attachment theory'... In Fairbairn's experience, analysing the Oedipus complex in his patients did not always lead to a resolution of their problems, and this dissatisfaction led him to develop the theory of schizoid phenomena. Fairbairn's first paper on this subject, 'Schizoid Factors in the Personality' (1940) was the beginning of an immensely innovative and creative period. It was this paper – in which Fairbairn coined the term 'schizoid' – that would later inspire Klein to alter her 'paranoid position' to 'paranoid-schizoid position', and that would similarly have a considerable impact on Donald Winnicott's thinking about schizoid states. This paper also marked the beginning of Fairbairn's pioneering thinking about borderline states, and their origins in the 'splitting' process, a defence against the pain of being rejected by insufficiently attentive parents .... He described the child splitting off the emotionally responsive side of his or her parents from the unresponsive side, thereby creating 'good' and 'bad' objects, and often also splitting the ego into 'good' and 'bad', a process often leading to borderline states. His development of a quite new theoretical and clinical approach to borderline states remains very important in the psychological treatment of such patients today.

In his first major paper, Fairbairn investigated schizoid factors in the personality:

> it becomes possible to recognize as essentially schizoid not only such phenomena as full-fledged depersonalization and derealization, but also relatively minor or transient disturbances of the reality-sense, e.g., feelings of 'artificiality' (whether referred to the self or the environment), experiences such as 'the plate-glass feeling', feelings of unfamiliarity with familiar persons or environmental settings, and feelings of familiarity with the unfamiliar. Allied to the sense of familiarity with the unfamiliar is the experience of 'déjà vu' – an interesting phenomenon which must likewise be regarded as involving a schizoid process. A similar view must be taken of such dissociative phenomena as somnambulism, the fugue, dual personality, and multiple personality. So far as the manifestations of dual and multiple personality are concerned, their essentially schizoid nature may be inferred from a discreet study of the numerous cases described by Janet, William James, and Morton Prince. And here it is apposite to remark that many of the cases described by Janet as

> manifesting the dissociative phenomena on the basis of which he formulated his classic concept of 'Hysteria' behaved suspiciously like schizophrenics – a fact which I interpret in support of the conclusion, which I have already reached on the basis of my own observations, that the personality of the hysteric invariably contains a schizoid factor in greater or lesser degree, however deeply this may be buried.
>
> *(Fairbairn, 1940, pp. 5–6)*

For Fairbairn, the schizoid was fundamental. Another Scottish analyst, Ronald Laing, followed Fairbairn in making the schizoid and schizoid phenomenon the centre of any explanatory system, as Marjorie Brierley explains.

> [Laing] … describes the existential-phenomenological foundations for a science of persons and the understanding of psychosis, leading to the conception of 'ontological insecurity' as the basic pathogenic experience, i.e., a feeling of insecurity instead of what we usually call 'safety of the self'. This may be due initially to inadequate 'mothering' (including not only lack of love, but treatment as a possession or 'chattel') and similar misfortunes in infancy and may be reinforced during later development by an unfavourable family set-up or other circumstances adverse to the growth of self-confidence or any feeling that it is safe and justifiable to be a person in one's own right …. Normally, physical birth is followed by 'existential' birth, i.e. the infant comes to feel 'real and alive and has a sense of being an entity, with continuity in time and a location in space'. Where 'this firm core of 'ontological security' is not acquired in infancy, future development is impaired by basic feelings of ontological insecurity. For a person with such shaky foundations 'the ordinary circumstances of everyday life constitute a continual and deadly threat'. 'If the individual cannot take the realness, aliveness, autonomy, and identity of himself and others for granted, then he has to become absorbed in contriving ways of trying to be real, of keeping himself or others alive, of preserving his identity, in efforts, as he will often put it, to prevent himself losing his self.' … It is not without significance that conclusions not incompatible with Laing's basic ontological insecurity have been reached by another psychotherapist. Guntrip, adopting Fairbairn's terminology, has recently suggested (Brit. J. med. Psychol. 1960, 33, 163) that 'we must recognize one further step in the process of ego-splitting as analyzed by Fairbairn, namely a split in the Libidinal Ego itself. … This represents the deepest split of all, of the Libidinal Ego into an active, masochistic, oral (anal and immature genital) Libidinal Ego and a passive Regressed Libidinal Ego. … the Regressed Libidinal Ego is the ego of profound schizoid, fear-driven retreat from life with its threats of depersonalization.'
>
> *(Brierley, 1961)*

Experiences of ontological insecurity are depicted throughout these films, but in particular in *Joker, You Were Never Really Here, First Reformed* and the *Revenant*, where it is depicted directly and one could argue that *ontological insecurity* could be used as the underlying condition depicted in *Us* and to explain the differences between Rick and Cliff in *Once Upon A Time In Hollywood* and between Matt and Alejandro, and Kate in *Sicario.*

Grotstein has described Fairbairn's theory of endopsychic structure as "the unsurpassed metapsychology of child abuse and of multiple personality" (Grotstein, 1991, p. 140) and "the most apposite paradigm yet proffered for child-abuse, child molestation, post-traumatic stress disorder and multiple personality disorder" (Grotstein, 1994, p. 123), all of which is directly relevant to the films we will be looking at.

Object Relationships

Object relationships are the atomic concept of Fairbairn's approach (Ogden, 1983; Padel, 1995). We experience the world through our relationships with others, and we learn through and from these relationships. We internalise and incorporate object relationships as the basis of the endopsychic structure that constitutes our personality. Freud in *On Narcissism* (1914) describes how relationships become incorporated and can then be used from one self / other position or another in accounting for anaclitic or homosexual object choice. In *The Ego and the Id* (1921) Freud argues that multiplicity, as in multiple personality disorder or dissociative identity disorder, could be understood as conflict between too many different internalised but unintegrated object relationships. Fairbairn produced a model of an ordered internal world based upon internalised object relationships that has developed over the life of the person but was originally laid down in the early years of that person's life. His psychology of dynamic structure has intrinsically personal components, ego structures and internal objects, as real as anyone in the external world. It is the activity of these internal objects and ego structures that grounds our relations to the world, and which reappear in our daydreams, phantasies, nightmares, dreams and art.

> ...my theory possesses all the features of an explanatory system enabling psychopathological and characterological phenomena of all kinds to be described in terms of patterns assumed by a complex of relationships between a variety of structures. It also possesses the advantage of enabling psychopathological symptoms to be explained directly in terms of structural conformations, and thus of doing justice to the unquestionable fact that, so far from being independent phenomena, symptoms are but expressions of the personality as a whole.
>
> *(Fairbairn, 1952, p. 129)*

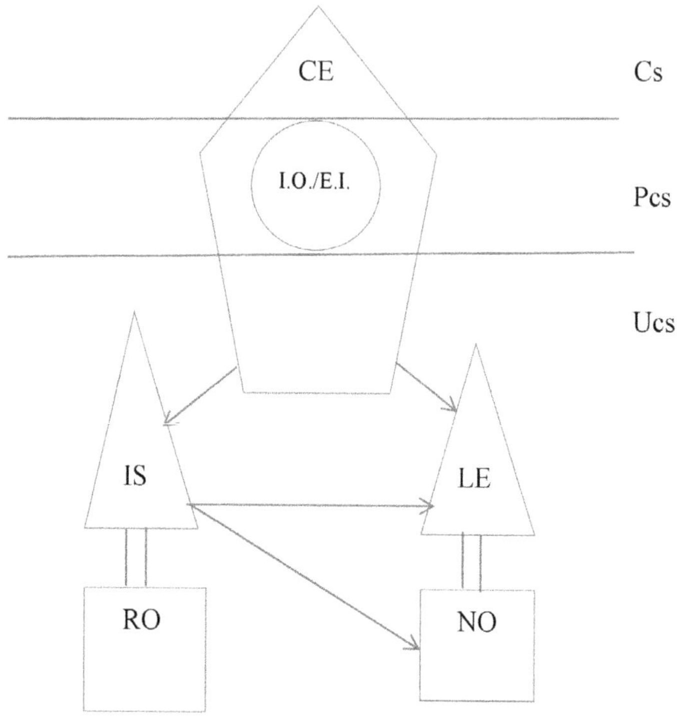

Based on Figure 1 from Fairbairn's 1944 paper.

The labels for the different dynamic endopsychic structures were later modified. In his 1954 paper on Hysterical States Fairbairn introduces the Antilibidinal Ego and Object and in his 1963 Synopsis of his theory he uses the following :-

In the Unconscious (Ucs) part of the mind :

> The Internal Saboteur (IS) became the Antilibidinal Ego.
> The Rejecting Object (RO) became the Antilibidinal Object.
> The Libidinal Ego (LE) remains the same throughout.
> The Needed Object (NO) becomes the Exciting Object (EO) in 1952 and then in later accounts the Libidinal Object (LO).

In the Preconscious (Pcs) part of the mind :

> He places the Ideal Object (I.O.)/Ego Ideal(E.I.) in the Preconscious (Pcs) part of the Central Ego (CE) [Author's addition to original diagram based upon the 1952 text.]

In the Conscious (Cs) part of the mind :

> The Central Ego (CE) remains the same throughout.
> The Central Ego or Self also contain Preconscious and Unconscious aspects which are part of the unrepressed, everyday, unconscious and preconscious, aspects of our internal world.

FIGURE 2.1 Fairbairn's model of endopsychic structure
Notes: CE, Central Ego; IS, Internal Saboteur; LE, Libidinal Ego; RO, Rejecting Object; NO, Needed Object; Cs, Conscious; Pcs, Preconscious; Ucs, Unconscious.

The full extent to which Fairbairn is committed to a model-based approach can be judged by the following (see Figure 2.1):

> the basic endopsychic situation … is by no means conceived as immutable from the economic standpoint. From the topographic standpoint, it must be regarded as relatively immutable, although … I conceive it as among the most important functions of psychoanalytical therapy (a) to reduce the split of the original ego by restoring to the central ego a maximum of the territories ceded to the libidinal ego and the internal saboteur, and (b) to bring the exciting object and the rejecting object so far as possible together within the sphere of influence of the central ego. The extent to which such changes can be effected appears, however, to be strictly limited. In its economic aspect, by contrast, the basic endopsychic situation is capable of very extensive modification … I conceive it as another of the chief aims of psychoanalytical therapy to reduce to a minimum (a) the attachment of the subsidiary egos to their respective associated objects, (b) the aggression of the central ego towards the subsidiary egos and their objects, and (c) the aggression of the internal saboteur towards the libidinal ego and its object. On the other hand, the basic endopsychic situation is undoubtedly capable of considerable modification in a psychopathological direction … I … suggest that corresponding to every distinguishable clinical state there is a characteristic pattern of the endopsychic situation … it must be stressed that the basic (and original) endopsychic situation is that which is found in hysterical states. I take the view that the earliest psychopathological symptoms to manifest themselves are hysterical in character; and I interpret the screaming fits of the infant in this sense.… although the basic endopsychic situation is the situation underlying hysterical states, it is itself the product of a split of the original ego, and is, therefore, a schizoid phenomenon. Thus, although the earliest psychopathological symptoms are hysterical, the earliest psychopathological process is schizoid. Repression itself is a schizoid process; and splitting of the ego is a universal phenomenon, although, of course, the degree of such splitting varies in different individuals. It is not to be inferred, however, that overt schizoid states are the earliest psychopathological states to develop. On the contrary, the earliest of such states are hysterical in nature. An actual schizoid state is a much later development – one which only materializes when the schizoid process is pushed to a point at which a massive repression of affect occurs and even an hysterical expression of affect is thereby precluded. Thus, it is only when a massive repression of affect occurs that the individual becomes unduly detached and experiences a pronounced sense of futility.
>
> *(Fairbairn, 1952, pp. 129–131)*

Through projective and introjective processes, characters in a film will give and take life from their counterpart in the endopsychic structure. Consequently, the external objects will be represented by different psychic structures. Thus, treating the film as if it were a dream involving the dynamics of various endopsychic structures is both natural and straightforward. Libidinal objects are specific, as are antilibidinal and ideal objects, and one can sustain contradictory beliefs about the various selves one maintains oneself to be by identifications with the various actors in the film. The overall dynamic then becomes important in that, the progressive integrative changes, within and between, the different structures represents a movement towards mature dependence, and the regressive disintegrative changes, within and between structures, a movement toward infantile dependence.

Endopsychic structure and the interpretation of dreams

During the 'Controversial Discussions' (King and Steiner, 1991), Fairbairn discussed Melanie Klein's conception of psychic reality and internal objects and commented,

> the explanatory concept of 'phantasy' has now been rendered obsolete by the concepts of 'psychical reality' and 'internal objects' which the work of Mrs Klein and her followers has done so much to develop; and in my opinion the time is now ripe for us to replace the concept of 'phantasy' by a concept of an 'inner reality' peopled by the Ego and its internal objects. These internal objects should be regarded as having an organized structure, an identity of their own, an endopsychic existence and an activity as real within the inner world as those of any objects in the outer world.
>
> *(Fairbairn in King and Steiner, 1991, pp. 358–361)*

In a seminal paper, Fairbairn (1944) describes how he derived his model of endopsychic structure from the dream of one of his patients. Fairbairn starts by describing his patient's dream.

> The (manifest) dream to which I refer consisted in a brief scene in which the dreamer saw the figure of herself being viciously attacked by a well-known actress in a venerable building which had belonged to her family for generations. Her husband was looking on; but he seemed quite helpless and quite incapable of protecting her. After delivering the attack the actress turned away and resumed playing a stage part, which, as seemed to be implied, she had momentarily set aside in order to deliver the attack by way of interlude. The dreamer then found herself gazing at the figure of herself lying bleeding on the floor; but, as she gazed, she noticed that this figure turned for an instant into that of a man. Thereafter the figure alternated between herself and this man until eventually she awoke in a state of acute anxiety.
>
> *(ibid., p. 76)*

Elaborating on his alternative to Freud's theory of dreams, Fairbairn says that, for him,

> after Freud's theory of psychical structure had become familiar, after Melanie Klein had elaborated the conceptions of psychical reality and internal objects and after I myself had become impressed by the prevalence and importance of schizoid phenomena, I tentatively formulated the view that all the figures appearing in dreams represented either parts of the dreamer's own personality … or else identifications on the part of the ego. A further development of this view was to the effect that dreams are essentially, not wish-fulfilments, but snapshots, or rather 'shorts' (in the cinematographic sense), of situations existing in inner reality … but, so far as the figures appearing in dreams are concerned … such figures represent either parts of the 'ego' or internalized objects. According to my present view, therefore, the situations depicted in dreams represent relationships existing between endopsychic structures; and the same applies to situations depicted in waking phantasies. This conclusion is the natural outcome of my theory of object-relationships taken in conjunction with a realization of the inescapable fact that internalized objects must be regarded as endopsychic structures if any theoretic significance whatever is to be attached to them.
>
> *(ibid., pp. 77–78)*

Fairbairn goes on to analyse the dream in the light of his views about endopsychic structure:

> In the manifest dream the actual drama involves four figures: – (1) the figure of the dreamer subjected to attack, (2) the man into whom this figure turns, and who then alternates with it, (3) the attacking actress, and (4) the dreamer's husband as a helpless onlooker. In our preoccupation with the actual drama, however, we must not forget our only witness of its occurrence – the dreamer herself, the observing ego. Including her, there are five figures to be reckoned with. At this juncture I venture to suggest that, if the dream had ended a few seconds earlier, there would only have been four figures, even on the assumption that the 'I' of the dream is considered; for it was only in the fifth act, so to speak, that a man began to alternate with the figure of the dreamer as the object of attack. This is an interesting reflection; for we must conclude that, up to the point of the emergence of this man, the object of attack was a composite figure. The special interest of this phenomenon resides in the fact that, as we have seen, there is good reason to regard a second figure as composite; for the attacking actress undoubtedly represented both another figure of the dreamer and the dreamer's mother. I venture, therefore, to hazard a further suggestion – that, if the dream had lasted a

> few seconds longer, there might well have been six figures, instead of five. It is safe, at any rate, to infer that there were six figures in the latent content; and this, after all, is what matters for purposes of interpretation. Assuming then that six figures are represented in the dream … our first observation is that the figures fall into two classes – ego structures and object structures. Interestingly enough there are three members of each class. The ego structures are (1) the observing ego or 'I', (2) the attacked ego, and (3) the attacking ego. The object structures are (1) the dreamer's husband as an observing object, (2) the attacked object, and (3) the attacking object. This leads us to make a second observation – that the ego structures naturally lend themselves to be paired off with the object structures. There are three such pairs: (1) the observing ego and the dreamer's husband, who also figured as an observer; (2) the attacking ego and the attacking object representing her mother, and (3) the attacked ego and the attacked object representing her father.
>
> *(ibid., p. 78)*

I have used this account to develop an approach to the interpretation of film using Fairbairn's theory of endopsychic structure and dreams. I have published or presented a number of papers on a Fairbairnian approach to interpreting film (1994, 2003a, 2003b, 2012, 2018), the main thrust of which is described below (p. xxx).

Using Fairbairn's object relations theory to interpret film

In Fairbairn's theory, the self, which is originally a bodily self, pristine and unstructured, develops into a highly structured and complex system of multiple object-relations based selves through natural and social development, whose overall long-term aim, as it develops to maturity, is to restore the integrity of the original self, reduce splitting as much as possible, and achieve coherence at a much more complex and sophisticated level than the original self.

In Fairbairn's model of endopsychic structure, a person is a system of selves and (internal) objects (which can also act as selves) in dynamic relationship, some conscious, some preconscious and some unconscious. The system, which comprises object relationships, grows and develops by incorporating or internalising, and projecting or externalising, and transforming object relationships. Whenever Fairbairn says object relationships, he means some affective relationship between a self and an object (person).

There is a *conscious* central self that interacts directly with the world; an ideal *preconscious* self which is composed of idealised object relations and acts like a conscience and an ideal self; an *unconscious* libidinal self which is composed of over exciting object relations and is repressed by the central self; and an *unconscious* antilibidinal self/internal saboteur, composed of over-rejecting object relations, which is also repressed by the central self. I believe there are also *preconscious* libidinal and antilibidinal object relations-based selves (Clarke 2005), which, together with the ideal self, form the normal range of object relational possibilities for the central self (see Figure 2.2).

When a person becomes involved in object relations with the outside world that stray beyond the overall expectations of their personality, then the unconscious libidinal and antilibidinal object relations can become activated, which invokes activity by the central and ideal selves to counteract this disturbance of expectations and restore order within the same, or a modified endopsychic structure.

Order can be restored directly by the central and ideal selves if they are able to repress the libidinal and or antilibidinal object relationships, otherwise a process of taking account of the disturbed state of inner reality has to take place. This might involve some initial reaction out onto the outside world, which needs to be acknowledged and assessed before any readjustments of the internal world are made, or, if it is a matter of ideas or images becoming conscious rather than being enacted, then some internal adjustments will be necessary.

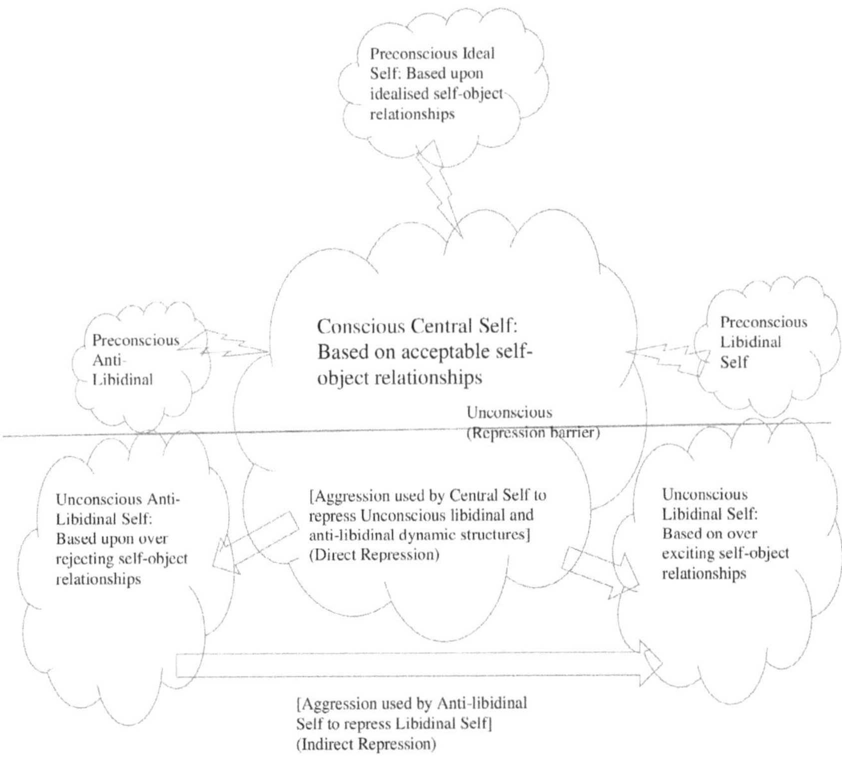

Based on Fairbairn's model of endopsychic structure, his 'psychology of dynamic structure', as described by the diagram in his paper Fairbairn, W.R.D. (1944).
(Amended to include preconscious libidinal and antilibidinal selves as per Clarke, G. (2005))

FIGURE 2.2 Fairbairn-based model of endopsychic structure

This can lead to changes in the inner world so that the ideal, central, libidinal and antilibidinal selves are altered. In some cases, this might be in order to expand the repertoire of object relations the person can tolerate (which suggests growth) and in other cases, in order to reduce or restrict the repertoire of object relations the person can tolerate (which suggests some limitation on their powers). The endopsychic structure is in a constant state of flux as the person negotiates the world.

When it comes to using this model to interpret film the first thing to do is to see which of the characters in the film might be the putative central self of the unfolding story and how that central self is being affected by events and objects (people) around them. Sometimes there will be more than one possible central self, which might eventually resolve into one self; or, multiple selves might form a coherent group, with a coherent personal identity. Sometimes the results of the disturbances to the central self's life can involve the destruction and loss of aspects of the functionality of the ideal and/or the central self. Sometimes this can be resisted and rejected, and the original status restored or improved.

The particular trajectory the overall story takes will have consequences for the viewer, thus the various genre – comedy, tragedy, farce, thriller or puzzle film, etc. – all involve different object relations and dynamics and elicit different sets of responses from viewers. Each of these different narrative forms will have an effect on the endopsychic structure of the central self and thus the viewer, to the degree that they identify themselves with the central self and the action of the film. The drama is the various changes undergone within and between the characters in the film.

As well as a possible central self I will also look for personifications of the other dynamic structures – the ideal self, the libidinal self and the antilibidinal self and note the dynamics between them. So, the drama of the film becomes the conflict between differently personified selves as dynamic structures. And because their associated objects also have a degree of autonomy these too will have personified representations in inner reality, and in the films, and form an essential part of the drama.

Fairbairn uses his model of endopsychic structure to describe and explain all of the significant aspects of psychoanalytic theory (Fairbairn, 1952, pp. 128–133; 1963) The development of the endopsychic structure starts with the incorporation of unsatisfactory object relationships into the infant's inner reality and produces an unstructured internal world of unsatisfactory object relationships, which form the basis of any subsequent schizoid developments. With the eruption of the teeth and the ability to direct aggression towards the (m)other, relations come to be regarded as either good or bad and the internal world begins to be structured by aggression used for repression. But, the ability to reliably direct aggression towards an appropriate bad object comes into question and the accidental possibility of directing aggression at the loved and needed other (the good object) can lead to depression. As experience with others develops, so too the internal world of good and bad object relationships becomes unwieldy and the need to control libidinal and aggressive responses becomes necessary. Fairbairn argues that at this early time in the development of the inner world the self becomes split into three experience-based dyads – acceptable self-object relations, over-exciting libidinal self-object relations and over-rejecting self-object relations. He also argues that an idealised version of the significant other is developed from the internalised acceptable object relations to become an ideal self and this ideal self comes to guide the central self, as it tries to control the unwanted or accidental activation of libidinal and antilibidinal object relationships based upon how the child responds to how it is being treated. Once this internal world is relatively stable this becomes the basic endopsychic structure and all future development of the self takes place by changes made to this internalised system of selves and internalised objects (object relationships). The development of a moral self occurs soon afterwards. As the child, under the influence of the ideal self, comes to regard aspects of himself as bad, rather than recognise that the needed good object (who has treated him badly) is bad. He thus avoids reacting to this treatment in a way that might threaten his wider attachment to the good object. Subsequently the ideal self, which is also a good self, can incorporate any good object relations experienced. A good (ideal) self advises a good-enough (acceptable) self on which bad (libidinal and antilibidinal) object relationships to activate in response to its experience of the world.

At this point in the child's development the activity of the endopsychic structure is complex but still by no means fully developed, no longer infantile as in the earliest period, but not yet sufficiently adult. Because the early object relations that went to develop the inner world were experienced when the child was still young there is room for learning, which will necessitate changes to the extent and disposition of the object relationships that constitute the internal world. The child enters a stage of partial independence where the different selves contribute differently to how the child responds to any situation. This is a period when the neuroses as defensive strategies may arise. These may arise in response to the need to overcome the infantile dependence on the significant other and begin to act independently and maturely. Fairbairn's account of this process analyses the technique used in terms of the way the internal objects are disposed and categorises the different neuroses as follows.

Obsession: The good (ideal) object is Internalised and the bad (libidinal and antilibidinal) objects are Internalised.
Paranoia: The good (ideal) object is Internalised and the bad (libidinal and antilibidinal) objects are Externalised.
Hysteria: The good (ideal) object is Externalised and the bad (libidinal and antilibidinal) objects are Internalised.
Phobia: The good (ideal) object is Externalised and the bad (libidinal and antilibidinal) objects are Externalised.

All of these neurotic responses are of variable likelihood and arise to accompany the process of trying to reliably establish objects externally in a realistic way, free of projection and introjection. These techniques can occur in succession as people struggle to establish themselves and their relationships on a mature footing. In general, the neuroses are defensive and are used to prevent a too rapid collapse of the person back towards infantile dependence. These techniques are centrally concerned with defining and establishing oneself as a separate person. In the Oedipus situation the child, through its experience of the actual parents, constitutes the Oedipus situation for itself. Having originally taken the mother or earliest caregiver as a template for the ideal, acceptable and bad objects, a similar process occurs with the father somewhat later so that there are then at least two ideal selves and objects, two acceptable selves and objects and two libidinal and antilibidinal selves and objects. In order to bring some clarity to the ever-burgeoning selves and internal objects a gendered identity is chosen in which one parent becomes the model for the ideal, the acceptable and the libidinal selves and the other gendered parent the model for the antilibidinal self. Because of the way this process develops, many of the object relationships with the dominant parent will have underlying relationships with the other parent hidden within them. A *maturely dependent* person is one who relates to properly differentiated others, people and situations, realistically for what they are without undue projection or introjection. This is the assumed goal of us all as we develop towards adulthood and maturity.

In 1994 in a paper developing an object relations approach to cinema (Clarke, 1994), I made the comment that the two positions that Klein developed, the 'paranoid-schizoid' and the 'depressive', could be used to categorise genre. I am repeating this here because it seems to be still relevant, although I would now read this in relation to Fairbairn's three developmental phases – infantile dependence, the quasi-independence of the transitional techniques and mature dependence respectively.

The paranoid-schizoid position, which is similar to and influenced by Fairbairn's ideas about the importance of the schizoid in earliest development, is characterised by splitting, projection, introjection and identification. However, Klein, as a child analyst, goes into far greater detail about the ways in which these processes are used, and appear, in protecting the child from anxiety. Attention is paid to the ways in which good and bad objects are internalised, manipulated, attacked, and so on, and how various body contents are expelled, projected and introjected. These feelings and their management are part of unconscious phantasy. It is important to note that they involve part-objects like the breast. Other aspects of the paranoid-schizoid position are omnipotence, magical thinking, primary narcissism and the symbolic equation or concrete thinking, as well as a terrifying punitive super-ego made of part-objects (male and female genitalia). In normal development, the paranoid-schizoid position or infantile dependence gives way to the depressive position sometime during the first year of life.

In the *tragic* aspects of the depressive position (Likierman, 1995) the child comes to realise that a lot of the 'bits and pieces' (part-objects) it has been loving, hating, consuming, rejecting, incorporating or attacking are in fact parts of one object – the mother (or primary caregiver). This brings with it the realisation that the child has been attacking and destroying its loved object. This in turn arouses anxiety and guilt about these attacks, fear that it has damaged the loved object, and, as a consequence, the need to make reparation. The consequences of the *moral* aspects of the depressive position are the recognition of others as separate and whole, containing both good and bad, recognition of the real world, and an ability for proper symbol formation and creativity. There is a transitional phase between these two positions called the *manic defence*, which seems to be more closely associated with the depressive position. In the manic defence, individuals protect themselves from depressive anxiety by excitement or laughter. Fairbairn has of course also specified a set of transitional techniques that lie between infantile and mature dependence.

Given the overall characteristics of these positions, and the fact that they represent a move towards greater morality with the achievement of the depressive position and the ability to direct love and hatred towards whole objects, an attempt to associate specific genre to particular positions can be outlined. All those films that deal with horror, torture, persecution, poison and similar themes would be associated with the paranoid-schizoid position. Similarly, all these films about war and the Wild West or similar, where the law of talion – an eye for an eye – dominates, would represent or reflect a paranoid-schizoid-position perspective, as would all films in which excessive killings, maimings, destruction, or fear of destruction are dominant. Given the nature of the super-ego in the paranoid-schizoid position as described by Klein, and the alien mother destroyer with obvious phallic overtones in *Alien*, this film could be seen as representing one woman's struggle to overcome the paranoid-schizoid position and enter the depressive position.

Comedies, comedy thrillers, romantic thrillers, thrillers without excessive killing, fantasy where excitement is the aim, would all seem to be representative of a *manic defence* against anxiety. I would expect them to have as part of their content serious issues of life and death, which they in some way or another undercut or defuse. Films that reflect the depressive position would contain deep, rounded, complex characters – real people – who lead lives that are believable and face problems that are both deeply felt and considered. The outcome of their lives might be tragic, but their attitude and courage would be exemplary. They would retain a creative approach to life, even if their times or circumstances were mean. Fairbairn's mature dependence would represent development beyond the *tragic* aspect of the depressive position to what Likierman describes as the *moral* aspects of the depressive position (Likierman, 1995) based in reparation or repair. What Fairbairn describes as *restitution* or restoration.

Absurdist comedy is closer to a paranoid-schizoid position where futility and the sense of annihilation are being defended against. Tragicomedy is closer to the depressive position, since it is a manic defence against depressive anxiety. Comedy itself appears to be transitional between the two positions, defending against the reality of either. It seems to be a way of protecting oneself from the limitations of either, and also a way of denying inner reality. What makes us laugh more than sincerities that can be punctured, or bodies as malfunctioning machines? Comedy acts to de-realise inner reality, imagine the unimaginable, invent new realities where reality is suspended; where space and time exist transformed, and bodies may become totally plastic; where the comedic players are immortal, always tilting at windmills, always popping back up after being knocked flat. They have hair-raising, neck-breaking, world-destroying roller-coaster rides through a world that is totally destroyed but remains untransformed.

Because films can and must engage inner reality, and because I would argue that inner reality is closer to an object-relations model of the sort I have described, the cross-cultural reception of films is not something that should surprise us, though it should surprise a cultural determinist. The detail with which different genres, and approaches within genres, can be attributed to particular positions, and nuances within those positions, probably depends upon our being able to expand and refine these positions along the lines Fairbairn indicates, and develop and combine the different modalities of defence in the transitional period – hysterical, phobic, obsessional and paranoid – and their characteristic ways of dealing with the accepted and rejected objects into the characterisation of genre.

It is worth noting that the combination of the paranoid-schizoid with the libidinal or over-exciting might be relabelled the polymorphous-perverse, which Freud identified as the psychosexual equivalent of infantile dependence. This suggests that the repression barrier is itself dynamic and the development of gendered positions as acceptable identities over recent time is a consequence of its being pushed deeper into what was called the infantile, and that repressive desublimation as a defence against the justified calls for sexual liberation, has led to greater freedom in one sense, but has bought with it a whole can of worms in the conundrum of what polymorphous perversity might deliver or whether it is the universal solvent of all difference and thus the harbinger of nihilism.

Fairbairn, Mature Dependence, and the Auteur

Fairbairn's developmental schema has three levels – infantile dependence (paranoid-schizoid), the quasi-independence of the transitional techniques (tragic depressive position) and mature dependence (moral depressive position). One question that could be broached is how one might characterise a film using Bazin's auteur theory by someone who has achieved mature dependence according to Fairbairn's theory?

In an extended essay in *Sight and Sound*, Bazin's approach is described as follows.

In one of his essays from the 40s Bazin projected that distant day when film studies would enter the university curriculum – and it was Bazin more than anyone else who played the role of midwife … In Bazin's view, it's this objective quality of the photograph – the fact that it is first of all a sensory datum and only later perhaps a work of art – which gives the medium its privileged relationship with the real. It follows that both photography and its spawn, the motion picture, have a special obligation towards reality. Their principal responsibility is to document the world before attempting to interpret or criticise it. For Bazin, this moral duty is ultimately a sacred one – the photographic media are, in effect, preordained to bear endless witness to the beauty of the cosmos … Photography and cinema, together with such innovations as colour stock, sound recording, anamorphic lenses and 3D, are successive responses to an obscurely planted desire for an ever more perfect approximation of the real … Bazin concedes that there is no art without artifice and that one must surrender a measure of reality in the process of translating it on to celluloid. The cinematic staging of the real can be carried out in untold ways, so it would be more suitable to speak of 'realisms' than of a single definitive realist mode. In this respect Bazin comes closer to endorsing the postmodern shibboleth of pluralism than his adversaries tend to realise – though he happily forgoes its nihilism … The crucial distinction for Bazin is … between, "Those directors who put their faith in the image and those who put their faith in reality." He took a notoriously dim view of … films made in the German expressionist style because he judged their elaborate manipulations of lighting and decor a wilful attempt to bend reality out of shape and force it to reflect perverse states of mind … What Bazin objected to in the work of Sergei Eisenstein was how the Soviet director splintered reality into a series of isolated shots, which he then reassembled through the art of montage … Bazin distrusted montage on the grounds that its dynamic juxtaposition of images hurtles the viewer along a predetermined path of attention, the aim being to construct a synthetic reality in support of a propagandist message …. Bazin valued those film artists who respected the mystery imbedded in creation … One such director was the Italian neorealist Vittorio De Sica, who … humbly renounced the hubristic display of authorial personality and thus enabled the audience to intuit the numinous significance of people and things …. Bazin recognised that film art always condenses, shapes and orders the reality it records, but what he looked for in filmmakers was a kind of spiritual disposition towards reality – an intention to serve it by a scrupulous effacement of means and a corresponding unwillingness to do violence to it through ideological abstraction or self-aggrandising technique … Given Bazin's passionate advocacy of this cinema of 'transparency', it may seem puzzling that he is likewise remembered in film history as an architect of the celebrated *politique des*

> *auteurs* ... If Bazin's criticism constitutes a cine-theology, it might almost be said that the auteur fulfils the role of saint – an inspired intercessor with reality. Bazin's stake in the *politique* can probably be traced back to his involvement in the 1930s Christian existential movement known as *personalism*, which posited the creative individual who takes risks, makes choices and exercises his or her God-given faculty of free will ... In the name of a higher realism, then, Bazin celebrated the long, uninterrupted take for its capacity to simulate the most elemental aspect of nature – its continuousness ... His great hero in this regard was Renoir, who, significantly for Bazin, combined long takes with the technique of deep-focus cinematography. Bazin considered this not just one aesthetic option among others but perhaps the very essence of modern cinematic realism. For him, the incalculable virtue of deep focus is its ambiguity. Since everything in the film frame can be seen with equal clarity, the audience has to decide for itself what is meaningful or interesting .... a possibility is nonetheless opened up that the viewer can... do the editing in his or her own head. In short, deep-focus cinematography invites an awareness of both personal freedom and ethical responsibility. In cinema as in life, we must be free to choose our own salvation ... It was perhaps impossible to avoid a head-on collision between Bazin's meditative humanism and a dogmatism that saw popular cinema as an ideological apparatus – an efficient machine for turning out docile citizens. As the most eminent critic of the preceding decade Bazin became a figurehead for the establishment and the militant new regime at *Cahiers* hammered him for his political complicity ... It must be admitted that his earnest belief in the intrinsically realist vocation of film puts him on the far side of postmodern relativism and doubt. Yet in so far as a compulsive scepticism and a jaded cynicism have become the orthodoxies of our age, this may be the moment to start rehabilitating reality – and André Bazin.
>
> *(Matthews, 2018)*

It is important to note that the ways in which Andre Bazin characterises films by an 'auteur' are consistent with the sort of films that you might expect from someone who is maturely dependent, in Fairbairn's terms. Bazin's normative view of the auteur, is based upon three premises which can, according to Sarris (1962),

> be visualised as three concentric circles: The outer circle as technique; the middle circle, personal style; and the inner circle, interior meaning. The corresponding roles of the director may be designated as those of a technician, a stylist, and an *auteur*.
>
> *(Sarris, 1962, p. 563)*

Films made from the maturely dependent position would be centrally concerned with interior meaning in Sarris's account, which he describes thus:

> The third and ultimate premise of the *auteur* theory is concerned with interior meaning, the ultimate glory of the cinema as an art. Interior meaning is extrapolated from the tension between the director's personality and his material. This conception of interior meaning comes close to what Astruc defines as *mise-en-scène*, but not quite. It is not quite the vision of the world a director projects nor quite his attitude towards life. It is ambiguous, in any literary sense, because part of it is embedded in the stuff of cinema and cannot be rendered in noncinematic terms. Truffaut has called it the temperature of the director on the set, and that is a close approximation of its professional aspect. Dare I come out and say what I think it to be is an *elan* of the soul.
>
> *(Sarris, 1962, pp. 562–563)*

It is worth reminding ourselves that the ego structures and internal objects of Fairbairn's theory which can appear to be static and thinly drawn are in fact complex constructions of multi-modal, dynamic personal structures which are under continual transformation.

A Fairbairnian Understanding of the Social Group

Carol Rovane (1998) introduced the concept of the 'group person' to understand multiplicity and the fact that a 'person' is not necessarily human sized but can be bigger or smaller – e.g., a group of human beings that comprise a person or a group of persons that comprise a human being. This latter is akin to Fairbairn's endopsychic structure but by no means the same. I think that Rovane's notion of a group person might be used to understand films like *The Seven Samurai, The Dirty Dozen, X-Men, Ocean's 11* etc. – any film involving a group of people unified by a common project and differentiated according to the function they serve within and for the group, but this is not being attempted here.

In-Group, Out-Group and Prejudice

Many of the films to be discussed involve conflict between different groups – affiliations with, and/or antagonisms towards – these groups. Given that prejudice in some form – racism, sexism, political affiliation, etc. – are also aspects of the films under discussion, a brief outline of Fairbairn's object relations understanding of the social group and the ways this has been used to understand prejudice by Ron Aviram (2007) are worth rehearsing. Fairbairn (1935) argues that Freud's two most outstanding contributions to a psychoanalytic understanding of sociology were:

1. His demonstration of the part played by aggression no less than libido within the economy of the individual mind and consequently in social life generally;

2. His demonstration of the influence upon human conduct of unconsciously accepted ideals, which have their origin in the reactions of the individual to his first social contacts, and which, during individual development, become organized into an internal psychical structure (the 'ego ideal' or 'super-ego') representing external social agencies.

(Fairbairn, 1952, p. 235)

For Fairbairn, all sociological developments must therefore be regarded as governed by two fundamental principles (c.f. Marcuse, 1969, *Eros and Civilization* and Freud, *Civilization and its Discontents*, p. 122):

1. The cohesion of social groups is a function of libido, and
2. The source of social disintegration in all social groups is to be found in aggression.

Reviewing the historical evolution of social groups Fairbairn describes the following developments as stemming from the original social group:

The Family, where the cohesion of the family depends upon libido being bound within the family and aggression being excluded from family relationships by the Oedipus situation. *The Clan*, although the clan embraces a number of families, it is itself organised as a family group characteristically ruled over by a chief, who represents the father of the clan, and to whom all members of the clan owe the allegiance of children to their father. The social cohesion of the clan is threatened by two dangers of an opposite kind: (a) the danger of the individual's libido being too much bound within the narrow limits of the family, (b) the danger of the individual's libido finding attachment outside the clan. The extension of exogamy to the clan carried with it, the risk of the individual's libido finding attachment outside the group; thus, leading in turn to the clan being superseded by: *The Tribe*, a union of clans. Like the clan, it is organised after the family model, being ruled over by a paramount chief whose authority is supported by religious sanctions. Exogamy is practised between the component clans; and in this way technical incest is avoided, while the necessity for marriage outside the tribe can be dispensed with. *The Nation*, evolved out of the tribe through a weakening of the influence of the clans comprised in the tribal organisation. This weakening of the clan influence within the tribe may be interpreted as due to the success achieved by the tribe in binding the libido of the individual to itself as a social group – a process aided by the establishment of tribal religious cults. The social cohesion of the tribe favours expansion at the expense of less stable communities.

Although the emergence of the nation as a social group involves the complete disappearance of the clan and the tribe, the family as a social group has hitherto resisted extinction during the course of social evolution. The survival of the family as a social institution shows that the nation has failed to eradicate the family group and has been compelled to come to terms with the family by incorporating it into the national organisation. According to psychoanalytical findings, a conflict arising out of the Oedipus situation characteristically plays a major role in the genesis of all psychopathological symptoms. It is less generally recognised, however, that the persistence of the Oedipus conflict in the unconscious of the adult involves the presence of two more specific conflicts:

1. The Oedipus conflict proper, i.e., a conflict arising strictly within the limits of the family system in the years of early childhood, during which the child's social horizon does not extend beyond the family circle.
2. A conflict arising out of the fact that intra-familial and extra-familial objects compete for the libido of the individual – a conflict arising characteristically during the adolescent period.

It should be noted that, while both these conflicts involve the question of loyalty to the patriarchal father, the latter represents the sociological conflict, in the individual, between the family system and more comprehensive social organisations such as the nation.

It is on the basis of Fairbairn's understanding of the development of groups that Aviram (2007) develops his account of in-group and out-group relations, a précis of which follows.

Given that Fairbairn's object relations theory provides a psychoanalytic developmental account of the relationship between early identification and adulthood identifications with social groups, then in Fairbairn's terms, *when infantile dependence persists into adulthood*, pathology can reflect boundary problems between self and other, and between self and group.

The recapitulation of primary identification can promote an over-identification between the person and his or her in-group. This suggests that the experience of self is overly dependent upon the evaluation of the group. When the in-group represents the self, perceptions of the in-group may need to be idealised, while the out-group is devalued. *The individual who has over-identified to compensate for developmental faults must rely upon collective identity to maintain a fantasy of power and safety.* Intrapsychically, the libidinal self wants to be attached to, and accepted by, the good idealised internal object. The antilibidinal self seeks to reject dependence upon a frustrating object by labelling it 'bad'. *Aggression is a response to the fear of losing love and security from the needed object, and the simultaneous inability to eliminate dependency on the 'bad object' due to unconsciously perceived attacks arising from internal objects leading to the need for self-defence.* This is achieved by projecting these bad objects outward and gaining a fantasy of safety, this process is reinforced by clinging to an idealised internal object, as well as by the development of the defence of avoiding the objects onto which the frightening figures have been projected. The cost of such a defence is a world that is filled with dreaded objects that restrict potential interactions. *Idealising the in-group and blurring the distinction between the self and the in-group can establish the fantasy of safety. Simultaneously, devaluing the out-group and its members is facilitated by the projection of bad objects* ... Out-group members who are discriminated against will tend to react negatively to the person or group that is the cause of mistreatment. For the overidentified individual, feared retaliation from out-group members can provide a conscious justification for his or her prejudice. Under this condition, both the hater and the hated are inextricably linked and help define each other. Anxiety stems from the danger aroused by the desire to reject the bad object that is simultaneously needed for one's identity and survival. The easiest solution to this problem is to use the intrapsychic mechanism of splitting – to love one object and hate the other. This identifies an important condition regarding the interdependence between an in-group and out-group. Both groups become interdependent for their self-definition and to distinguish between the idealised and good self/group, and the devalued bad other/group (based on Aviram, 2007, pp. 10–13).

Aviram's account illustrates the way in which our failure to achieve *mature dependence* and remaining at the level of *infantile dependence* can contribute to distortions of in-group and out-group identifications and the dynamics of prejudice. We anticipate finding these processes active in a number of the films to be reviewed. In particular, the failure to achieve the highest level of social integration, i.e., a national ideal and identity, means that the whole (social) system fractures and 'tribes' of identity-based groups proliferate, all potentially opposed to one another to some degree. This is clearly the case in *The Revenant*, which is about nation-building and *Widows*, which is about local politics and the absence of a unifying narrative, and *Sicario*, which is full of in-groups and out-groups at war with each other. It is clearly true of *Us*, which is about deep divisions and prejudice across the nation. It is an important part of *Joker* and *You Were Never Here*, which are about the damage done to individuals in a 'dog eat dog' neoliberal environment. *First Reformed* is about the lack of a unifying narrative over climate change, which encourages dissociation and atomisation. In *Roma*, it is about the class and Indigenous-based stratification of society. In *Once upon a Time in Hollywood* it is about the response to the post-war boredom and uptight mentality of the 1950s being overturned by youth culture and the advent of the Hippies and reactions against them in the 1960s.

References

Aviram, R. B. (2007) 'Object Relations and Prejudice: From In-group Favoritism to Out-group Hatred'. *International Journal of Applied Psychoanalysis Studies* 4 (1): 4–14.

Aviram, R. B. (2018) 'A surprising cause of prejudice'. *Psychology Today*, 22 Jan. https://www.psychologytoday.com/us/blog/contemporary-psychoanalysis-in-action/201801/surprising-cause-prejudice (last accessed Aug 2020).

Bion, W. R. (1962) *Learning from Experience.* London: Tavistock.

Brierley, M. (1961) 'Review of: *The Divided Self. A Study of Sanity and Madness*: By R. D. Laing. (Studies in Existential Analysis and Phenomenology). (London: Tavistock). (1961)'. *International Journal of Psycho-Analysis*, 42: 288–291.

Britton, R. (2021) *Sex, Death and the Superego*, 2nd edition. London: Routledge.

Burton, E. S. (2016) https://psychoanalysis.org.uk/our-authors-and-theorists/ronald-fairbairn, (last accessed 16 Jan 2020). Excerpted from the British Psychoanalytic Society web page on Ronald Fairbairn.

Callenbach, E. (1975) *Ecotopia*. Banyan Tree Books.

Clarke, G. (1994) 'Notes towards an object-relations approach to cinema'. *Free Associations*, 4 (3): 369–390.

Clarke, G. S. (2003a) 'L.A. Confidential: object relations and psychic growth', *British Journal of Psychotherapy* (March).

Clarke, G. S. (2003b) '*The Piano Teacher: object relations and psychic disintegration*', presented at the 'Culture and the Unconscious' conference at School of Oriental and African Studies, London, July 2003.

Clarke, G. (2005) 'The preconscious and psychic change in Fairbairn's model of mind'. *International Journal of Psychoanalysis*, 86 (1): 61–77.

Clarke, G. S. (2012) 'Failures of the "moral defence" in the films *Shutter Island, Inception* and *Memento*: Narcissism or schizoid personality disorder?' *International Journal of Psychoanalysis*, 93 (1): 203–218.

Clarke, G. S. (2018) 'Trauma, dissociation and time distortion in some "puzzle" films.' *Thinking through Fairbairn: Exploring the object relation model of mind* (pp.119–146). London: Routledge.

Fairbairn, W. R. D. (1935) 'The Sociological Significance of Communism Considered in the Light of Psychoanalysis'. In Fairbairn W.R.D. (1952) *Psychoanalytic Studies of the Personality* (pp. 233–246). London: Routledge.

Fairbairn, W. R. D. (1940) 'Schizoid Factors in the Personality.' In *Psychoanalytic Studies of the Personality* (pp. 3–27). London: Tavistock.

Fairbairn, W. R. D. (1941) 'A Revised Psychopathology of the Psychoses and Psychoneuroses'. *International Journal of Psychoanalysis*, 22: 250–279.

Fairbairn, W. R. D. (1944) 'Endopsychic Structure Considered in Terms of Object-Relationships'. *International Journal of Psychoanalysis*, 25: 70–92.

Fairbairn, W. R. D. (1952) *Psychoanalytic Studies of the Personality.* London: Tavistock.

Fairbairn, W. R. D. (1955) 'Observations in Defence of the Object-Relations Theory of the Personality'. *British Journal of Medical Psychology*, 27 (2–3): 144–156.

Fairbairn, W. R. D. (1963) 'Synopsis of an object-relations theory of the personality'. *International Journal of Psychoanalysis*, 44: 224–225.

Gammage, B. (2012) *The Biggest Estate on Earth: How Aborigines Made Australia.* London: Allen Unwin.

Gillespie, P. (2018) 'Neoliberalism of the seamier side of psychoanalysis'. www.apres-coup.org/mt/archives/subject/City2018/Gillespie.pdf (last accessed 8 Mar 2020).

Glover, E. (1932) *On the Early Development of the Mind.* London: Imago.

Grotstein, J. S. (1991) [Review.] 'Hughes, J. M. Reshaping the Psychoanalytic Domain: The Work of Melanie Klein, W. R. D. Fairbairn, and D. W. Winnicott'. *Psychoanalytic Quarterly*, 60: 136–140.

Grotstein, J. S. (1994) 'Notes on Fairbairn's metapsychology'. In J. S. Grotstein and D. B. Rinsley (eds.), *Fairbairn and the Origins of Object Relations Theory* (pp. 112–142). New York: Guilford.

Hall, S., Massey. D., Rustin, M. (2015) *After Neoliberalism? The Kilburn Manifesto*. London: Lawrence and Wishart.
Jameson, F. (2016) *An American Utopia: Dual Power and the Universal Army*. London: Verso.
King, P. and Steiner, R., eds. (1991) *The Freud-Klein Controversies 1941–1945*. London: Routledge.
Layton, L. (2013) 'Psychoanalysis and Politics: Historicising Subjectivity'. *Mens Sana Monogr*, 11: 68–81.
Layton, L. (2014a) 'Some psychic effects of neoliberalism: Narcissism, disavowal, perversion.' *Psychoanalysis, Culture & Society*, 19: 161–178.
Layton, L. (2014b) 'Grandiosity, Neoliberalism, and Neoconservatism'. *Psychoanalytic Inquiry*, 34 (5): 463–474.
Likierman, M. (1995) 'Loss of the Loved Object: Tragic and Moral Motifs in Melanie Klein's Concept of the Depressive Position'. *British Journal of Psychotherapy*, 12 (2): 147–159.
Marcuse (1969) *Eros and Civilization*. London: Sphere Books.
Matthews, P. (2018 originally published 1999) 'Divining the real: the leaps of faith in André Bazin's film criticism'. https://www2.bfi.org.uk/news-opinion/sight-sound-magazine/features/andre-bazin-divining-real-film-criticism-overview.
Ogden, T. H. (1983) 'The Concept of Internal Object Relations'. *International Journal of Psychoanalysis*, 64: 227–241.
Padel, J. (1985) 'Ego in Current Thinking'. *International Review of Psychoanalysis*, 12: 273–283.
Rovane, C. (1998) *The Bounds of Agency: An Essay in Revisionary Metaphysics*, London: Princeton University Press.
Rustin, M. (2013) 'A relational society'. In *The Kilburn Manifesto*. Surroundings.
Sarris, A. (1962) 'Notes on the auteur theory in 1962'. *Film Culture* (Winter 1962–1963), 27: 1–8.
Scharff, C. (2016) 'The Psychic Life of Neoliberalism: Mapping the Contours of Entrepreneurial Subjectivity'. *Theory, Culture & Society*, 33 (6): 107–122.

3

THE REVENANT (IÑÁRRITU, 2015)

The Past is Another Country

Internal Worlds

Applying Fairbairn's theory to the story

There is one obvious candidate for the *Central Self* and that is frontiersman, Glass (Leonardo Di Caprio), about whom the whole story revolves. He is opposed, attacked, and put into jeopardy by trapper Fitzgerald (Tom Hardy), a 'freebooter', interested only in how much profit he can make, who is thus a prime candidate for being an Antilibidinal *Self / Internal Saboteur*. In charge of the trapping expedition is an American Captain (Domhnall Gleeson) representing the current nominal rulers of the country as they set up forts and gradually colonise the whole of the native American territory. Ostensibly committed to honour and fairness, he represents a form of conscience or *Ideal Self*. Behind all this lies the chief of a native American (Pawnee) tribe Elk Dog (Duane Howard), whose daughter Powaqa has been abducted and abused by the French military who are also laying claim to the territory as a French colony. This is the native Americans' land which has been taken over and is being exploited unmercifully by the colonists, French and American. The Indian Nation was the highest level of coherent sustainable social organisation on the continent before the colonists came to conquer and exploit it. They might have represented the *Ideal Self* before the colonists arrived, and Glass is closely associated with their ethos through his native American family. The French military groups who are trying to lay claim to the same border territory are happy to trade with the native Americans to thwart the American troops with whom they are in competition for overall control of this rich territory. These can also be seen as *Antilibidinal Selves / Internal Saboteurs*.

DOI: 10.4324/9781003206224-4

Glass has lived with Pawnees, married into a tribe and had a son by his Pawnee wife. He values and respects his adopted native American heritage. His wife has been killed in a raid on an Indian village by French soldiers (Žižek in one of his YouTube lectures says that his friends among 'native Americans' prefer the non-PC term 'Indians' because it speaks volumes of the white man's ignorance and stupidity.) His young son has been saved from the attack and is nursed back from near-death by Glass's loving attention. Glass has subsequently made a living as a guide for the various expeditions into the wilderness, mainly for furs, usually protected by the American military. Glass's son Hawk, now adolescent, accompanies him and they work together as a team. Their current job is to guide a group of trappers from the fort to a productive area for fur hunting. While they are preparing and collecting the pelts for transfer back to the fort, a group of Pawnees attack them and steal as many of the pelts as they can find. With the whole party on the run and the Indians hard on their heels, the captain asks Glass to recommend the best way to get back to the fort. Fitzgerald opposes all of the advice that Glass offers on the grounds that he might lose some of his anticipated profit from the expedition. After some discussion, the Captain pulls rank and supports Glass's suggestion, so they stash the pelts and start off across country through the mountains back towards the fort.

Meanwhile, the Pawnee chief is trading with the French, using the pelts they have taken from the trappers. The Chief argues with the leader of the French who is prepared to trade guns and ammunition for pelts, but not the horses that the chief insists upon. The French leader says that they had an agreement, and the Indians have to honour it. It turns out that the Chief does understand, and replies in French, outraged at the French leader talking about honour. The French leader objects to the fact that the pelts have already been branded and will fetch less. The Chief points out that they have stolen everything from the Indians, the land, the animals, their livelihood. Earlier we have seen the pyramidal piles of bleached Buffalo skulls. The Chief continues to complain about two white men who sneaked into the village and kidnapped his daughter Powaqa. He says he will leave the French the pelts because honour demands it but that he will take the horses to help find his daughter. He says they are free to try and stop them if they like.

These colonists are destroying an ecologically aware, sustainable culture and the ecosystem it supports and is supported by, for fur-related trinkets and other fetishized commodities.

After the first day's march towards the fort, the trappers set up camp, and while scouting out the camp Glass disturbs a mother bear and her two cubs. The bear attacks Glass and mauls him viciously. Glass manages to kill the bear with a shotgun and a knife, despite being terribly wounded. The rest of the troop try to help minister to his wounds, with the captain sewing him back up as best he can while Fitzgerald leads the call to leave Glass, who he thinks is going to die anyway and get back to the fort as quickly as possible to preserve their (Fitzgerald's) earnings. The Captain resists this logic and they make a stretcher for Glass and try to carry on. As they enter the mountains there is a change for the worse in the weather. The Captain, encouraged by Fitzgerald, considers putting Glass 'out of his misery', as they weigh up the pros and cons of continuing onwards, but he cannot summon the courage to do it. He asks for volunteers to stay behind and look after Glass and makes the offer attractive by saying that there will be a reward for their help when they reach the fort. While the two other men, his son Hawk and Sam, are not doing it for the money and say so, Fitzgerald is, so it isn't surprising to find him plotting to kill Glass later and trying to get Glass to agree to his killing him, so he can have a defensible position.

Fitzgerald kills Hawk and tricks Sam into thinking they are under attack and must leave immediately and that Glass is already dead anyway. Sam is concerned that they didn't bury Glass properly but is bullied into doing what Fitzgerald wants him to do anyway. Fitzgerald takes them along by the river to get back to the fort, a route that Glass warned against because of the native Americans knowing and probably following that route.

Glass, when he regains consciousness and finds his son's dead body, realises what has happened and after grieving he begins to crawl his way out from where they are and back towards the fort. Slowly he makes his way down to the river and starts following it.

Sometime after he has left the camp where Hawk was killed, the native American tribe searching for both more pelts and for the chief's daughter find the camp where Fitzgerald abandoned Glass. They set off after Glass and arrive at the river soon after Glass, who has to use all his guile to avoid them. Whilst trying to hide at the base of a cliff Glass gets swept down the river over rapids and, using a tree trunk to cling on to, is swept along to a relative safe location well downstream.

Glass makes it back to the fort sometime after Fitzgerald, but both the Captain and Fitzgerald have been alerted to the fact Glass is still alive by the arrival of a starving French soldier carrying the water bottle that Sam left with Glass.

The native American group, the chief reunited with his daughter thanks to Glass, only reappear at the end of the film to despatch Fitzgerald, who has been in a fight with Glass, having killed the Captain a little earlier.

Identity

> Fairbairn (1935) recognised that the original social group is established in the family. He suggested that as we develop relationships with the surrounding community the available groupings substitute for the original identification with our parents. Given that this is a developmental process we can speculate that the original identifications influence subsequent identifications with individuals and social groups ... We can extrapolate further by suggesting that early

> familial identifications are recapitulated during early adulthood … and provide a template for identifications with in-groups.
>
> (*Aviram, 2007, p. 6*)

I want to look at the way Glass's identity is deeply connected to the native American tribal life he adopted, his native American wife who was murdered by a soldier, and his son who is murdered by Fitzgerald, and which murder is the impetus and scourge driving Glass on to wreak his revenge upon Fitzgerald.

> Fairbairn's theory suggests that if primary identification persists into adulthood and dependence needs are directed beyond the family, primary identification with these parental substitutes would minimize differentiation between self and group … When little or no differentiation is present between self and group, then overidentification with the group would provide an emotional experience of self. Under these conditions the in-group represents the self.
>
> (*op. cit.*)

In Glass's dream, depicted at the beginning of the film before the titles, we are presented with his attachment to his wife and child and a resolute and courageous attitude towards all setbacks. These do not just appear at the beginning of the film but reappear throughout the film. In particular, when Glass is struggling for survival, he draws upon these internalised figures to help him get through the terrible situation he is in, even though he knows that both the people on which these internalised figures are based, are dead. They are internalised good objects in his ideal self.

> Fairbairn (1935) suggested that there was a close link between the self / individual and the social world and proposed that the first social group into which we are born is the family. He asserted that we obtain our identity from the psychodynamics of the family constellation, and this normally involves the development of emotional ties which later become templates for emotional attachment to others in adulthood. He further suggested that the community and the in-group become substitutes for the original family group, and early attachment patterns are also later repeated in subsequent social identifications with social groups.
>
> (*Knight, 2015, p. 466*)

There are two main messages that can be taken from the words and images used to represent the dreams and phantasies Glass is having as he struggles to survive and avenge his son's murder. One is about endurance and persistence as an active process, not giving up and relying on the assistance of others, about the need to fight for existence. The second is about the hidden deep power at the core of us all, reflected in the durability of the trunk of the tree even if its branches are torn off and damaged. At the end of the film, he is still being encouraged onwards by the hallucinated image of his wife, his ideal object, his lover.

The reparative key to his overall journey is his ability to give up his vengeful ideas at the very end, and to practise what the Pawnee who helped him survive advises. His heart is bleeding but he leaves revenge in the hands of the creator.

Native American

There are a number of significant scenes in the film which represent aspects of Glass's internal world through memory, dream and phantasy and all are accompanied by dialogue in the Pawnee language, accessible to us through subtitles but not accessible to most of the other characters in the film.

At the beginning of the film, before the titles appear, we are focused on Glass living with his native American wife and son aged about five. They are all asleep in a native American tent-like structure. There is a voiceover which is Glass speaking the native American dialect and talking to his son initially. Glass tells his son that he knows that he wants the impending suffering to be over.

We then enter the dream visually, as well as aurally, and see Glass's wife and son standing out in a strong wind near a tree, enjoying being blown about as Glass enters the shot, telling them he is with them. We see images of his wife and son laughing as they are being blown about by the wind. He continues, admonishing them not to give up. There is an image of their tent on fire, the fire having been started deliberately by a soldier. Glass urges them to keep breathing and not give up. This is followed by an image of Glass sitting on the ground, nursing his son, surrounded by the devastated native American village in flames urging his son to breath, and to keep breathing. This strand of the dialogue refers to a situation depicted later, after the native American village has been attacked and burnt by soldiers, and after Glass's wife has been killed, where Glass is trying to keep his traumatised son alive by drip-feeding him water from a sopping wet rag. Glass has become the nurturing mother encouraging his son, with all his might, to fight, to live.

These two strands of the dream, the visual and the aural, are incomplete and they are added to as the film continues. We later discover that Glass's wife has been shot dead by a soldier and that Glass killed the soldier. We also discover that Glass spent a lot of time nursing Hawk, his son, and getting him to recover from the trauma of the raid on their village and the death of his mother. This is all also work on his inner world, coming to terms with the loss and keeping these internal objects alive to him in vital ways.

Later in the film more details of the raid return to the delirious Glass while Hawk nurses him. Their roles are reversed. Hawk asks him if he can hear the wind and if he remembers what his mother used to say about the wind and its inability to defeat a tree with a secure base. Hawk then repeats phrases that

Glass used when nursing him after his mother's murder, encouraging him to keep breathings and acknowledging how much he misses her.

This gives way to an image of Glass and his wife, forehead to forehead in deep communion, a sort of primal couple, which changes to one of Hawk carrying a live bird on his wrist in the village, followed by the village itself, now a burning ruin, and Glass nursing Hawk and giving him water from a wet rag. As he nurtures Hawk, he reassures him that he is by his side and encourages him to keep breathing and to fight to stay alive. We then hear his wife talking about the tree in a storm and sheltering near it. Hawk then sees his mother being shot by a soldier. Hawk talks about looking at the branches of the tree and fearing that it must fall. Glass sees his dead wife. As she lies on the floor a small bird representing her spirit or soul appears from the wound in her chest and flies away. Hawk resumes his account of the tree and its uncanny stability, followed by an image of his wife in front of a tree and Glass cuddling Hawk as they sleep. The words and images represent the deep attachment there is between Glass and his internal objects – his wife and their son – his in-group.

Later, Glass is helped by a lone native American in much the same situation as he is – alone and starving, but who has just shot a buffalo. Glass appeals for help and food and is given both. Glass tells him that he has been injured by a bear and deserted by his men who also killed his son. The Pawnee tells him that he has lost his family too, that the Sioux killed them and that he is going south to find more of his people. He says that his heart is bleeding but he knows that revenge is in the creator's hands.

The Pawnee, aware of how ill Glass is from the bear attack, unselfishly spends time and effort building a sweat lodge and preparing unguent from herbs to dress Glass's wounds. As the sweat lodge is being built, Glass's wife's words appear on the soundtrack again as Glass stirs back to semi-consciousness. He remembers her talking again about how in a storm when you stand in front of a tree you might think that it will fall if you just look at the branches but that if you look at the trunk you will see how stable it is. This represents an appeal to his own resilience and inner strength and the power of their group identity.

While he is recovering in the sweat lodge, Glass has a vision-dream of being in a dilapidated church with religious murals and a bell teetering above him. He sees Hawk and they embrace, but when he breaks the embrace, he finds he has been hugging a tree. But this contact with Hawk is also an indication that he is healing, absorbing some of the youthful vigour of his son into his own body. When Glass eventually revives, he discovers that the native American has gone but left him food and water and that his body and mind is much healed by the treatment he has been given.

At the end of the film, Glass's wife appears to him again and seems to be leading him onwards like a guardian angel.

Death and rebirth

Since one meaning of 'revenant' is 'to return from the dead' it is not surprising to find a variety of situations that could be interpreted as a return to a womb-like situation, followed by a rebirth from this womb. The most obvious and striking of these is how Glass survives a blizzard after he and his horse have plummeted from a cliff while being chased by the native Americans. His horse is killed in the fall, but he is not, another example of his mysterious power of survival. He can see that there is a blizzard coming so he eviscerates his horse, takes off his clothes and climbs inside the horse's carcass to protect himself from the storm. Similar events previously have included his being put into a shallow grave and half covered with earth, followed by a heavy snowfall from which he drags himself, having been deserted by Fitzgerald and Sam. Earlier, he 'holed up' in a small cave by the river, and later he is placed in the sweat lodge, which is also covered by deep snow before he recovers enough to emerge. While trying to get back to the fort after heavy snow he builds himself a snow cave and scrawls on the wall a condemnation of Fitzgerald for killing his son. Each of these return and rebirth cycles sees him becoming stronger and are often accompanied by a flashback, or phantasy, based upon his experience of living with the native Americans and more importantly his experiences with his wife and child.

Central self

The obvious contender for the *Central Self* is Glass, since we follow him throughout and he is clearly the main subject of the overall story being told. If there were other contenders, they would be Fitzgerald and the Captain, but both of these are unsuitable since we don't focus on their stories to anything like the extent we do Glass's story. The Captain does act as a potential central self in that he is involved in organising and running the hunting expedition with a mixture of soldiers from the fort and professional trappers. Glass is their guide because of his extensive experience of these border lands, once the established home of native American tribes, and currently disputed by American and French colonial administrations seeking to gain the various riches the territory holds, by force if necessary. Glass, as *Central Self*, goes from living with a tribe of Native Americans to losing his wife to a colonial raid and later to the death of his son at the hands of Fitzgerald. This leads on to his being abandoned to his fate by the expeditionary party and to his surviving, as much by luck as judgement, and the help of another native American who he meets on the way back to the fort. It is the memory of his wife and child as aspects of his *Libidinal* and *Ideal Selves* that sustains him and spurs him on to persevere in his journey and seek revenge for Fitzgerald's murder of his son Hawk.

Antilibidinal self (Internal saboteur)

The obvious candidate for the role of the *Antilibidinal Self* is Fitzgerald. Fairbairn's original title for this dynamic structure was the 'internal saboteur' which perhaps, more exactly, fits Fitzgerald since throughout the film Fitzgerald is constantly agitating, arguing, intervening against Glass and his advice in order to try to maximise his own profit and achieve his own ends at any cost. He is an icon of fiercely individualistic, totally self-interested, neoliberal economic mankind. He is constantly trying to gain favour for his plans and denigrates all other plans, especially Glass's plans. When he judges that the Captain has opened the way to his getting some money for looking after Glass, whom he has no sincere intention of actually helping to survive, he volunteers to help and calculates that he can recoup some of what he has lost on the pelts. He bullies Sam into lying to support the story he tells about leaving Glass after he 'died' and thus qualifying for the bonus the Captain offered. Fitzgerald is out for himself and prepared to use whatever tricks he can to achieve his own ends even at the expense of someone else. He even tries to win at the very end when he is fighting Glass in the snow on the banks of the river. When it is clear that Glass has won the physical battle between them Fitzgerald once again raises the idea there was a deal between them. The deal Fitzgerald proposes was for Glass to blink to indicate he is happy for Fitzgerald to kill him and help Hawk get back to the Fort, a disingenuous promise at best. Glass denies he ever assented to the deal despite the fact that in great pain and terribly wounded he at last lets his eyelids fall momentarily while fighting to maintain them open. Glass reasserts that there was no deal, and that Fitzgerald killed his boy in cold blood. Fitzgerald taunts Glass that he has come all this way for a revenge that he will never be able to enjoy because there is nothing that will bring his boy back to him. The Internal Saboteur attacks the self-confidence and the memories of Glass in order to undermine him.

Glass rehearses the words in Pawnee from the earlier encounter with the native American who helped him, as he pushes Fitzgerald into the river, acknowledging that revenge is in the hands of the creator now. The Chief and his daughter and a small party of native Americans are approaching. They kill and scalp Fitzgerald and send his carcass off down the river, leaving Glass to go free.

Libidinal and Ideal selves

The best candidates for the *Libidinal* and *Ideal selves* are Glass's native American wife and their son. They are both dead well before the end of the film but, as described earlier, have been present as part of his deep self throughout. It is in their honour and with their encouragement and on their behalf that he has persisted, survived against the odds to avenge the killing of their son and the earlier killing of his wife.

Having completed the redemptive, reparative and restorative task of seeing both his son's and his wife's death avenged and having relied upon the words of his wife about the durability of a deeply rooted tree throughout to sustain him, as he struggles to climb up out of the river valley and return to the fort, he hallucinates his wife again, going ahead of him and waiting until he can start climbing too, to keep up with her. The last shot of the film is of him turning to look at the camera as he prepares to renew his ascent.

External Worlds

A political future? A violent past

While it is clear that Glass with his deep experience and understanding of both the colonial and the Indigenous culture (Indian Nation) is the best candidate for the central self, it is equally clear that Fitzgerald as antilibidinal ego is a more appropriate model for the development of the American nation as it has become known to us. A rapacious appetite for fetishistic pleasure and the accumulation of money, capitalist greed and exploitation, a no-holds-barred, winner-takes-all approach is characteristic of entrepreneurs like Fitzgerald. The Captain represent the rule-bound lineaments of duty to whoever is in charge, essentially conservative forces blindly imposing the status quo. Glass is the face of a possible future that was never realised, while Fitzgerald represents rampant capitalism kept in check to a degree by the conservative forces of the status quo in the person of the Captain. The 'Indian Nation' was potentially the best and most sustainable accommodation to the American environment possible at the time, but it was crushed and hounded by capitalist greed, commodity fetishism and ideological myopia.

In the beginning ...

It is worth considering the more or less contemporary accounts of the developing American state and its view of the Indigenous peoples. While the action of the film is set circa 1823, the movement towards excluding the Indian Nation from any political power was already well advanced, as Andrew Jackson's 1829 inaugural address to Congress bears witness.

> Our conduct toward these people is deeply interesting to our national character. Their present condition, contrasted with what they once were, makes a most powerful appeal to our sympathies. Our ancestors found them the uncontrolled possessors of these vast regions. By persuasion and force they have been made to retire from river to river and from mountain to mountain, until some of the tribes have become extinct and others have left but remnants to preserve for a while their once terrible names.
>
> *(Jackson, 1829)*

Discussing the subsequent, commentators on Tocqueville, McQueen and Hendrix warn against an easy slippage into a language of "Indian nomadism and easy American expansionism" since as subsequent scholars have made clear, "American territorial expansion was a complex and contentious political project, in which institutions were mobilized to create the 'empty' spaces that white American citizens would then fill."

> Discourses of nomadism and inevitable Indian extinction were essential to this project and were contested by tribes and their allies. The United States did not, as conventional American Political Development (APD) accounts have often suggested, expand easily and naturally to its current territorial and political shape. Its expansion was often the result of systematic and contested choices made by political actors.
>
> *(McQueen and Hendrix, 2017, p. 672)*

There is an antique flavour to the main arguments for rejecting the Indian Nations as civilised and as Nations. This is based upon the fact that the Indians are nomadic hunter gatherers and the whites are agriculturalists. Hunter gatherers follow the animals and plants they depend upon and have little use for boundaries and ownership. A hunter gatherer is forever an earlier and less sophisticated form of society for Tocqueville and his contemporaries. Because of their 'outmoded' form of social organisation, they are 'doomed to extinction'.

> Like many of his Jacksonian American contemporaries, Tocqueville invokes "nomadism" not only as the "wandering" ways of Indians, but also as a set of natural and inescapable dispositions that prevent them from "settling," civilizing, and adapting to the conditions of democratic modernity. Claims about Indian nomadism were central to Jacksonian defenses of Indian removal, and many elements of Tocqueville's text reflect these discourses.
>
> *(ibid., p. 664)*

As De Tocqueville himself writes in 1830 with heavy irony:

> The conduct of the Americans of the United States toward the natives … breathes the purest love of forms and legality. Provided that the Indians stay in the savage state, the Americans do not mix at all in their affairs and treat them as independent peoples; they do not permit themselves to occupy their lands without having duly acquired them by means of a contract; and if by chance an Indian nation can no longer live on its territory, they take it like a brother by the hand and lead it to die outside the country of its fathers …
>
> *(De Tocqueville, 2002, pp. 334–335)*

In their introduction to *Democracy in America*, Mansfield and Winthrop write:

> Tocqueville's account of the plight of the Indians chillingly brings to light the ease and hypocrisy with which majority tyranny comes to be exercised in the New World. Anglo-Americans, motivated not by ill will, much less by racial hatred or prejudice, but merely by greed and contempt, not only denied native Americans their rights, but were well on their way to exterminating them "with marvelous facility – tranquilly, legally, philanthropically, without spilling blood, without violating a single one of the great principles of morality in the eyes of the world" … The Anglo-Americans … destroyed the wild game on which the Indians lived, thereby driving them from their traditional hunting grounds and leaving them to face death at nature's hand. They contemptuously dismissed the Indians' appeals to justice and common humanity.
>
> *(De Tocqueville, 2002, pp. 47–48)*

McQueen and Hendrix (p. 668) describe the main sleight of hand revealed by Tocqeuville's analysis as follows:

> In the providentialist strands of Tocqueville's text, it is the Indian's *inherent* and insurmountable nomadism that prevents him from being included in the American *demos* … Yet Tocqueville also calls attention to a nomadism of retreat, which is induced by both the actions of individual Anglo-Americans seeking Indian lands and the policies of the Jacksonian state. This kind of movement has profound effects on the character of Indian tribes. It creates a more severe form of "barbarism" by which Indians become even more unrooted than before. Tocqueville explains the results of these displacements in stark terms: "Europeans, after scattering the Indian tribes far into the wilderness, *condemned them to a wandering and restless life*, full of inexpressible miseries." … Here, nomadism is an *artifact*, rather than a natural disposition. (Emphasis in original)

As we shall see, this nomadism as artifact is central to *Nomadland*, a retreat in that case from the harsh reality of neoliberalism and urban decay by the old and working poor.

It is interesting to note that the social opposition between these two modes of production which is assumed to have developed at the origins of the so-called agricultural revolution about 10,000 years ago in the Middle East rears its head again during times of colonisation and later. True of Africa, America and Australia, it is also interesting to note that recent scholarship (Gammage, 2012) has suggested that the Australian Aborigine had been ecologically and sustainably managing the whole of the flora and fauna of the Australian continent for thousands of years whilst remaining predominantly hunter gatherers.

A classic example of the Marxist adage that "social being determines consciousness" can be found in Turnball's famous, or infamous, *The Mountain People* (1966) about the Ik, a hunter gatherer society forced to become agriculturists.

> forbidden by the Ugandan government to hunt game in the Kidepo National Park [they] are compelled to farm and forage for food in the barren mountain heights ... Drought and starvation have made them a strange and heartless people, mistrustful of their own kind.
>
> *(Turnball, 1972, cover material)*

This is in stark contrast to Turnball's account of hunter gatherers, based in his work on the Mbuti, described in *The Forest People* (1966):

> ...hunters frequently display those characteristics that we find so admirable in man: kindness, generosity, consideration, affection, honesty, hospitality, compassion, charity and others ... For the hunter in his tiny close-knit society, these are necessities for survival; without them society would collapse ...
>
> *(Turnball, 1972, 31)*

An examination of twenty-first-century nomadism ends this book (Oscar winner *Nomadland*) and the Trump era, but as we shall see, America cannot go home by returning to the road. The origin story of the nation as writ large in *The Revenant* is one of destruction and disrespect toward nature and the indigenous peoples of America. The roots of 'the Dream' are sown inextricably into the violent death of another way of life. That of the Native American and their way of life, holistic, at one with nature and bending to its will. To a large degree too it is also built on the backs of the slaves forcibly brought across the Atlantic from Africa.

For Iñárritu, communing with the dead, acknowledging the past, is a kind of redemption. In his earlier film *Biutiful* (2010) the protagonist Uxbal, literally on his death bed, finds some peace with his father in a vision in the snow and with his living daughter by passing on a family ring to her. Nature features in the form of elements (the wind, the water) and animals – an owl (in *The Revenant* it is a Hawk). His father gave the ring in question to his mother before he left Spain. He explains that she was pregnant, and she never saw him again.

Like Glass himself, it is clear then Uxbal's father was a frontiersman. Earlier in *Biutiful*, when he worries about his impending death and the fate of his children without him, his best friend reassures him that the Universe will look after them. In much the same way, in *The Revenant*, the Pawnee tells Glass that revenge is in the creator's hands.

At the end of *The Revenant*, like *Biutiful*, we return to the world of ghosts, a dream world of the dead. Images are reversed. We go from the water to

Glass's face at the end – the reverse is true at the beginning of the film. In the opening lines of the film, we hear Glass's memory of his wife and child and his use of these internal figures as resources that will encourage him to go on breathing as long as he can, that he must fight for breath, that he must endure. As Glass looks at us, we are left looking into him. Wondering how long he will live? Whether and how revenge has brought him closer to his son or not?

Glass stands in for America and its dreams – what might have been. In his struggle with Fitzgerald, we see an America borne out of extreme violence against Indigenous people and nature and the use of the law of the talion. We wonder how long Glass's America will in fact sustain itself and 'keep breathing'.

The past is indeed another country, one that predates these settlers and frontiersmen and their American Dreams. The Native Americans are clearly in tune with the natural world; indeed, they did do things very differently here.

References

Aviram, R. B. (2007) 'Object Relations and Prejudice: From In-group Favoritism to Out-group Hatred'. *International Journal of Applied Psychoanalytical Studies*, 4 (6).

De Tocqueville, A. (2002) *Democracy in America*. Translated and edited by H. C. Mansfield and D. Winthrop. Chicago and London: University of Chicago Press.

Gammage, B. (2012) *Biggest Estate on Earth: How the Aborigines made Australia*. Sydney, Melbourne, Auckland and London: Allan & Unwin.

Jackson, A. (1829) 'Address to Congress, Dec. 8, 1829'. In *Documents of United States Indian Policy*, 3rd edition. Lincoln: University of Nebraska Press.

Knight, Z. G. (2015) 'The Self in Prejudice'. *South Africa Journal of Psychology in Africa*, 25 (5): 461–469.

McQueen, A. and Hendrix, B. A. (2017) 'Tocqueville in Jacksonian Context: American Expansionism and Discourses of American Indian Nomadism in *Democracy in America*'. *American Political Science Association*, 15 (3) (September).

Turnball, C. (1966) *The Mountain People*. London: Eyre and Spottiswood.

Turnball, C. (1972) *The Forest People*. London: Simon and Schuster.

4

ROMA (CUARÓN, 2018)

Anamorphic Social Realism

Internal Worlds

Introduction

As the very useful and informative Netflix documentary called "The Road to Roma", about the making of the film, based upon an extensive interview with Cuarón argues, the film is a painfully realistic portrayal of Mexico City circa 1970 in the upper-middle-class home of a doctor and his family. It is a deeply autobiographical film about a period in Cuarón's own childhood and young manhood and a tribute to the part played within the household by their Indigenous (Mixtec) maid (Manita / Cleo), who supported the family materially and emotionally throughout this turbulent period in their history and in the history of Mexico. It is her life as an example of *Mature Dependence* that interests me here in particular. There is a dedication to the real maid at the end of the film.

Politically, there are two significant dates referenced by Cuarón in the documentary, 2 October 1968 and 10 June 1971, the first being an attempt to restore democracy that failed, despite garnering some middle-class sympathy, and the second an attempt to reclaim democracy, which became a bloody massacre thanks to the Halcones, an unofficial paramilitary force. Manita / Cleo and the grandmother of the family both witness the massacre from a furniture shop window, where Cleo has been taken to buy a cot for her unborn baby. A group of Halcones chase a man into the shop and shoot him. Cleo recognises one of the gang as the man who got her pregnant and then abandoned her and denied all responsibility for her or the baby, a martial arts fanatic. He threatens her and the grandmother with a pistol before running off. This trauma leads to her waters breaking and her going

DOI: 10.4324/9781003206224-5

into labour and, despite the best efforts of all involved at the maternity ward, her losing the baby, which is stillborn.

Towards the end of the film Cleo saves the two youngest children, Pepe and Sofi, from drowning despite being unable to swim herself, and her role as the emotional centre of the family is graphically revealed as she, the children's mother and the four children huddle together on the beach. They are all incredibly grateful for what Cleo did and the mother tells her how much they all love her, which leads to Clio confessing, while she is distraught, her guilt at having not wanted her child to be born, which, at this moment of maximum emotional intensity, she confesses to them all as they surround and support her, enfolding her in their love.

Throughout we see the world from the Indigenous maid's perspective, which allows for the whole of the society and culture to be laid out before us in much the way that both Brecht and Lukács, despite their differences, recommended as the basis of something like socialist realism in the arts, of which this seems exemplary to me.

> According to this conception of art as a mode of reflection, the function of a work of art is to present humans with the totality of the objective, historical reality within an "homogeneous medium" ... The employment of such a medium makes it possible for art to single out and represent the universal aspects of a given form of human reality as a "closed world-in-itself" or as an "intensive totality" ... As Lukács argues ... the medium of each specific form of art establishes strict laws that allow the work of art to adequately present the whole world of humanity from a specific standpoint. For this reason, such works of art allow us to comprehend the universal aspects of our existence and to consciously participate in the collective life of humanity ... This effect of art Lukács describes as "defetishization" ... anticipating the ethical demand of overcoming alienation that he formulates in the *Ontology*. A successful work of art can thus have the effect of "catharsis" ... transforming the "whole person" of everyday life (the person who is entangled in their diverse relationships) into a "person as a whole" (the person who realizes their humanity by acquiring a sense of self-consciousness regarding the richness of human relations that constitute the historical development of humankind).
>
> *(Stahl, 2018, section 4.4 Aesthetics)*

For Bertolt Brecht, the dramatic structure underlying any situation reflects the structure of social forces at work in society. Since Brecht was a Marxist living in an industrial capitalist nation, he understood these social forces as competing classes (although he also dealt with historical struggles, such as 'science versus church,' in his play Galileo). For Brecht, any narrative either disguises and obscures the structure of social forces or reveals and exposes them. Brecht's drama aims to reveal and expose the social forces underlying everyday events.

(Brecht, 2016, March 25)

Brecht's theater is realistic, although not in conventional terms. Realism, Brecht writes, lays bare society's causal network. The realistic writer shows that the dominant viewpoint is the viewpoint of the dominators; he writes from the standpoint of the class that has prepared the broadest solutions for the most pressing problems afflicting human society – that is, from the standpoint of the proletariat. Realism, as Brecht understands it, is a Marxist critique of society. His anti-illusionist theater depicts the social problems of his age. Brecht argues that literature should give the working masses a truthful representation of life.

(Brecht, 2019, May 4)

Story

The story is of a professional middle-class Mexican household circa 1970, a loving recreation of the house and family that the director, Cuarón, was born into and lived among, including the staff that shared their home. It focuses on the life and experience of their indigenous maid called Manita/Cleo in this film.

The household is divided, as was the norm, between the family – mother, father and grandmother of Spanish origins – and their four children, all in the latency period of development, "the stage of personality development, extending from about four or five years of age to the beginning of puberty, during which sexual urges appear to lie dormant" (Latency period: Dictionary.com). After Oedipus, and before puberty, three boys and a girl, who is the second youngest. They have two Mixtec maids who do all of the household chores – cleaning, cooking, serving, washing up, washing, ironing, fetching and carrying, as well as a good proportion of the childcare of the four children; and an Indigenous chauffeur and handyman. They also have a dog that shits freely all over the courtyard/driveway which separates the house from the neighbouring houses, that is partly enclosed but open to the sky. This area where the dog shits freely is the responsibility of the maids to clear up with a brush and a bucket and wash down using some cleaning products. It becomes a focus for complaint by 'the man of the house' on the day he leaves the family despite the efforts to which the Mixtec maids have gone to clear up and disinfect the area.

The film opens with one of the maids cleaning down the courtyard, after which the family start to return from school and work. Manita / Cleo is depended upon by all of the family to provide food and sustenance and to minister to their emotional needs too.

We follow the life of Manita / Cleo the Indigenous maid, who is also the main childcare support for the children, overseeing their going to bed and getting up, their breakfast and dinner and bedtime. The two younger children in particular clearly loving and depending upon her for emotional support.

Early in the film we observe a nervy and tense morning as 'the man of the house', a doctor at the local hospital is apparently leaving for a conference in Ottawa, Canada, with his wife showing more anxiety and distress than would be normal. This turns out to also be the doctor leaving home to live with his mistress, a fact that is kept from the children until towards the end of the film.

Mature dependence

Perhaps the most difficult idea in Fairbairn's theory is that of *Mature Dependence.* Whilst it has similarities to Freud's genital position it is aspects of relationality rather than the erotogenic aspects that are to the forefront for Fairbairn. In the schema for the development from *Infantile Dependence* to *Mature Dependence, Infantile Dependence* is characterised predominantly by an attitude of *taking* and objects are all internalised, while the stage of *Mature Dependence* is characterised predominantly by an attitude of *giving* and the objects are all externalised. These two stages are separated by a transitional stage of quasi-independence as the person develops from infantile to mature dependence (Fairbairn, 1952, p. 39).

> *Mature Dependence* – 'mature dependence' rather than 'independence', since a capacity for relationships necessarily implies dependence of some sort. What distinguishes mature dependence from infantile dependence is that it is characterized neither by a one-sided attitude of incorporation nor by an attitude of primary emotional identification. On the contrary, it is characterized by a capacity on the part of a differentiated individual for co-operative relationships with differentiated objects. So far as the *appropriate biological object* is concerned, the relationship, is, of course, genital; but it is a relationship involving evenly matched giving and taking between two differentiated individuals who are mutually dependent, and between whom there is no disparity of dependence. Further, the relationship is characterized by an absence of primary identification and an absence of incorporation.
>
> *(Fairbairn, 1952, p. 145, emphasis in original)*

Cleo / Manita is, from my perspective, someone who is maturely dependent and behaves in a loving and giving way throughout, even in circumstances in which we can become enraged on her behalf, as with the treatment she receives from Firmín, her boyfriend who is a member of the paramilitary Halcones. He gets her pregnant and then makes himself scarce when she tells him that her period is late. Later on, he quite deliberately frightens and threatens her when she finds out where he is and goes to see him and tells him she is pregnant, and it is his baby. When Manita tracks Firmín down he is at a training camp for the Halcones on a playing field where the initials of President Echeverría are prominently displayed.

> President Echeverría took office in December 1970. Before, as interior minister – the nation's internal security chief – he oversaw the violent suppression of student protesters in the late 1960's … On his watch, government forces killed scores of people. The most notorious killings – the Tlatelolco massacre, named for the neighbourhood in which it happened – took place just before the 1968 Olympics in Mexico City. As president, Mr. Echeverría appointed Fernando Gutiérrez Barrios, who had been chief of Mexico's fearsome secret police, as deputy interior minister. Mr. Gutiérrez Barrios, who died in 2000, was adept at recruiting undergraduates to infiltrate left-wing groups, paying their tuition in exchange for information … His campus recruits were usually the children of PRI stalwarts. They formed the ranks of a government strike force created to counter the student movement in September 1968, days before the Tlatelolco killings. It was called the Falcons – Halcones, in Spanish … In May 1971, the student movement began to stir again. In Mexico City, thousands began to plan a demonstration, set for June 10. Contemporary evidence, including cables from the United States Embassy in Mexico City after the attacks, established that President Echeverría supported the Falcons and their attacks … The United States Embassy in Mexico City was well aware of the group. On Jan. 6, 1971, it sent a cable to Washington saying a prominent Mexican Army colonel, Daz Escobar, had come to the embassy seeking training for a group of young army officers and university students. The cable described the students as likely government infiltrators of campus organizations. Washington granted the request, though no American-trained Falcons took part in the killings on June 10, 1971… A subsequent cable from the American Embassy noted, "It is well established that the Halcones are an officially financed, organized, trained and armed repressive group, the main purpose of which since its founding in September 1968 has been the control of leftist and anti-government students."
>
> (New York Times, *1971*)

Firmín asks Manita why she is there, and she tells him that she has been trying to find him because she is pregnant, and it is his baby. He becomes aggressive and denies that he is the father and warns her that if she persists in saying this then he will beat the shit out if her and her baby. He tells her to go away and never look for him again, whilst threatening her with some violent martial arts moves before dismissing her as a fucking servant and trotting off to join other paramilitaries on the back of a truck taking them to Mexico City.

Firmín represents an *Antilibidinal Self / Internal Saboteur* and is involved in the Corpus Christi Massacre:

> On June 10, 1971, in the vicinity of the Meritorious National Teachers School, students from the National Autonomous University of Mexico (UNAM) and from the National Polytechnic Institute (IPN) took over the streets to demand then-President Luis Echeverría (1970–1976) political freedom and the democratization of teaching in support of students in Monterrey … It was the first large student protest after the events that took place three years before in Tlatelolco, one of the most painful imprints in Mexican history … The peaceful protest that was carried out at the Mexico-Tacuba Road, turned into a massacre after the irruption of the paramilitary force "Los Halcones" (The Hawks), which opened fire to repress the students, which left at least 22 killed, several missing, and 50 injured … This massacre is considered one of the most violent episodes of the government's "dirty war" against opposing political movements by the late 70s and early 80s …. The episode is known as "El Halconazo" or "The Corpus Christi Massacre" and is portrayed in Alfonso Cuarón's "Roma."
>
> *(https://www.eluniversal.com.mx/english/1971-corpus-christi-student-massacre-one-bloodiest-chapters-mexicos-history)*

Mixtec: Values and beliefs

The brief resume of Mixtec values and beliefs below, reveals the parallels there are between Mixtec beliefs and an object relations approach, the highest point of which is *Mature Dependence*, characterised as an attitude of giving which throws light on the attitude that Manita / Cleo has taken from her culture.

> The Mixtec have an ancient, extremely rich and complex spiritual life. Many of these beliefs continue to exist, in syncretic fashion, alongside Roman Catholicism and, increasingly evangelical Christian faiths, with no apparent contradictions. According to traditional Mixtec belief, all things, living or inanimate have a spirit (also known as animism) … Failing to acknowledge someone is not only considered rude, it characterizes the individual, literally, as an ignorant brute as the Mixtec ascribe certain types of behaviors to animals, others to humans … The Mixtec, like many other peoples of Oaxaca, embrace the concept of mutual or reciprocal help. *Da'an* is a Mixtec word akin to the meaning to offering or gift. It is appropriate to provide the host of a large party, for example, with a *da'an* of several cases of beer or soft drinks. *Tequio* is service to the community, and traditionally is required of all male members. *Tequio* is taken extremely seriously; even those who have migrated to other parts of Mexico, or the United States are expected to return home to meet this obligation. It is becoming somewhat more common for women who remain at home to fulfil this service.
>
> *(Mixtec.org, Jan 2021)*

Recognition

There are throughout the film examples of the way that the maid and her feelings are ignored or minimised, despite the overall recognition of her supreme importance to the household at the end of the film after the mother and her four children all appreciate that, even whilst wrestling with her grief and guilt over the stillbirth of her baby girl, Cleo was prepared to risk her life to save the lives of Sofi and Paco.

Early on, on the evening of the day before the doctor deserts his family, he complains loudly about the dog shit and the untidy refrigerator, both of which fall within the domain of the maid's responsibilities, but which contrast with the complete lack of any contribution to the overall maintenance of the house by anyone other than the maids. After the emotional departure of the husband, the wife unloads her resentment at her husband by telling the maid off about the dog shit.

The mother and grandmother of the children are liberal about accepting the maid's pregnancy and getting her appropriate furniture and continuing to employ her, but when the maid, despite her trying, cannot prevent Paco from witnessing his mother's phone call about her distress at the husband leaving them, all the bad feelings are again projected onto the maid. But the maid's carry out all of the childcare and housework and are constantly running around, often quite literally, working and in the case of the husband going to a conference, moving cases from car to home and vice versa.

There is one telling moment when the mother, deserted by her husband, comes back one evening, drunk, and drives their oversized American car against the walls, totter's unsteadily up to the very pregnant Cleo, takes her face in her hands and says, "We are alone", then giggles to herself, "No matter what they tell you. We women are always alone." This contrasts to some degree with their experience at the hacienda they go to for Christmas with a number of other families and their staff, where Cleo and the other Indigenous servants seem to have some degree of solidarity among them. The depiction of the very different living conditions between the rich 'white' population of Spanish origin and the 'black' population of Indigenous population is polarised between middle-class wealth and excess and working- or under-class poverty and lack of basic services, both publicly and privately. The genteel suburb in which they live versus the shanty town, unmade flooded roads, duck boards, etc. of Cleo and the suburbs of her class. From their experience of the village near the hacienda, which reminds Cleo of her home village where there is a degree of agriculture, animal husbandry and well-being, which is better off than the suburbs, the other maid tell Cleo that her mother's house has been taken over, but Cleo is unable to go home to help, as she is pregnant and her mother would be ashamed and perhaps lose face among her neighbours.

The maid, like servants in general, also sees and hears a lot more than other members of the family – she knows about the separation, she sees the father with another woman when she and the children are on their way to the cinema. She is also privy to the fantasies of the youngest child who seems to be dreaming or fantasizing that he has lived both earlier and later than the current time. As she is helping him get ready for school, he talks about their relationship in the following way.

Pepe says that when he was old that she, Cleo, was someone else. Cleo asks him if he meant when he was old or when he gets old, and Pepe says that it is when he is old. When Cleo asks when this was, he says that this was before he was born. She asks him what he did then, and he says he was a fighter pilot. She asks him if he liked being a fighter pilot and he says no, he didn't: it was scary.

Their conversation is brought to a conclusion since Cleo has to leave to help the husband pack.

Towards the end of the film, as they are going swimming, Pepe starts telling Cleo that, when he was older, he used to be a sailor. But he then recounts how he drowned in a storm. He remembers that the waves were huge, that it was dark, that there was lightning, and that he didn't know how to swim.

The two younger children love and trust Cleo, and she is there to comfort and contain them as they comfort and contain her, while she guiltily confesses to not having wanted her stillborn child.

External Worlds

Alfonso Cuarón

Alfonso Cuarón is one of a trio of contemporary Mexican directors whose careers can be described as extraordinary. Cuarón, along with Alejandro González Iñárritu (as discussed above in *The Revenant*, Chapter 3) and Guillermo del Toro, the 'three amigos' as they have been dubbed, dominated the Oscars for a decade with five of the last directing Oscars going to the three of them, and their films picking up a huge number of awards and success around the world. Like Iñárritu, whose Oscar-winning VR work *Carne y arena (Flesh and Sand*, 2017) stands as one of the great works on migrations in the twenty-first century, Cuarón's most personal work is about his home country, and about the impacts of globalisation on ordinary people.

Cuarón has made three important personal films – *Roma, Y Tu Mamá También* (2001) and *Children of Men* (2006). Roma clearly links back to the other two – it opens with two question mark images. What is that wave of water on the tiles? Where is that plane going in the sky? Later we learn, *Roma*'s antagonist lives in the dirt and mud, city earthquakes shake its hospitals and a fire engulfs its centre. Huge waves sweep its protagonists towards the film's denouement. Like his compatriot Iñárritu's *The Revenant* and *Biutiful, Roma* is a powerful elemental film and a film about the precariousness of being a parent.

We begin with this wave of water, as Cleo literally begins to clean the shit off the yard floor of the middle-class compound-home she lives and works in. The house is in Roma – the affluent area of Mexico City that alongside Condessa represents wealth and success in Mexico, as well as being Cuarón's real-life neighbourhood growing up.

The water that opens the film is part of a repeating motif in *Roma* (the cleaning, the premature breaking of Cleo's amniotic waters and the waves that nearly drown her and the children) that loops back to the end of *Children of Men*. That film ends on waves of hope. The anti-hero Theo dies on the English Channel, as he delivers Kee and her baby to the Tomorrow project, finally finding some kind of redemption for himself and perhaps the human race.

Children of Men

Cuarón represents different parts of his country's histories in all three films, and all three are road movies of a sort. Whilst *Roma* draws on road movie elements, circling back to the gated family house at its centre, *Y Tu Mamá También* is clearly an homage both to American road movies and the French New Wave, set against the huge changes in Mexican politics at the end of the twentieth century. *Children of Men* is another genre movie, a dystopian sci-fi of sorts, whose entire second half is also a road movie – one of pursuit and escape from London to the English Channel. Cuarón acknowledged that he made *Children of Men* post-9/11 to try to understand the coming twenty-first century, and in doing so realised he had to bring the unruly mess of Mexico City to London. This is part of the ongoing neoliberal *Brazilification* of the West, a neologism Douglas Coupland (1991) first coined as "*The widening gulf between the rich and the poor and the accompanying disappearance of the middle classes.*" The end point of this Brazilification is the "gated compound" life of the wealthy and the lawless favelas seen in cities like Rio and Cape Town and Mexico City.

In Cuarón's brutal vision, this is imported to London and mixed in with a populist xenophobic society (prescient of Trump and Brexit). This is of course part of the world allegorised in *Us*, a world of the dispossessed, and this Brazilification can be clearly seen in America today. In LA, a huge homeless population (in excess of 60,000 people night-to-night in LA County – (Scott, 2020)) live in tent cities near, or even in, the affluent areas of Beverly Hills and Santa Monica, and this has now spilled into the billionaire hippy homes of Dennis Hopper's old Dogtown home Venice Beach (Lowe, 2021). Homelessness is the coal face of capitalism, a living, growing symptom of the new American Nightmare.

Cuarón creates a whole world of the future in *Children of Men*, something he emulates by equally creating a whole world of the past in *Roma*. The detail of both worlds is astonishing. It is true that in 2020 if you wanted to understand our present moment best – Covid, Trump, Brexit, the ongoing aftermath of Middle Eastern wars; you need look no further than *Children of Men*. Flisfeder (2017, p. 160) says it "provides for us a kind of cognitive mapping of our potential future, should things continue unchanged." As Horvat (2018) puts it when discussing *Children of Men* with the director, "*the older it gets, the newer it is. Either way you know, at that time when I watched it – it was 2006, it was as if it was a movie from the future about our dystopian future*". In *Roma*, the reverse seems true: is this film from a dystopian past about our own present? Undoubtedly, post-9/11 and 2008, neoliberal, Western economies, through a series of shocks and austerity, both deliberate and unplanned, have become Brazilified. 2020 Mexico City and London or LA are closer than ever, in every sense. Considered together, *Roma* and *Children of Men* take us back to our future present.

There is one stylistic link in form and intention that goes beyond these thematic similarities, however. Simple plot and genre descriptions fail to really enunciate *what* these films are, why they are so successful at what they do and why they are such incredible examples of pure cinema. Cuarón is an auteur in that he elevates his own material through complex *mise-en-scène*. He understands cinematic spectacle in an old new way – a mixing of generic styles if you like. It is as if he takes the scale of *Ben Hur* and mixes it with the documentary or social realist style of *Bicycle Thieves*. Perhaps the title *Roma* is a nod to the Italian neorealist style established in De Sica's Roman classic or even the classic Rossellini work, *Rome – Open City*.

The background is the foreground

Roma, like the other films, is a small intimate story told on a huge canvas. What Žižek (a huge fan of *Children of Men* and a contributor to the Criterion collection DVD documentary accompanying the film – *The Possibility of Hope*) labels an *anamorphic* view. Others including the Breathing Frames channel (2016) and Mariel Calloway (2014) highlight this style as "*the background is the foreground*".

The anamorphic lens is a very cinematic wide lens favoured most recently by cineastes such as Nolan, P.T. Anderson and Tarantino, and these lenses are used today to create a cinematic effect. They are double the width of normal spherical lenses and give a slightly curved effect at the edges – they are considered more cinematic, especially in an age where most films are shot digitally.

The effect is clear. In Cuarón's triptych of films the camera is often moving sideways, but always with this wide-angle anamorphic view. Sometimes the camera 'roves', leaving the protagonist's side (or behind) to carry on and follow what would traditionally be called 'background' action. Even when the camera is still in *Roma* (as it is in the house initially or during Cleo's visit to the cinema for instance), the action around and behind the protagonists is hugely detailed and richer than almost all dramatic films, particularly today. It is as if Cuarón has recreated the entire world of Mexico City in that period. Wolmart (2017) brilliantly describes the camera movement as "tethered", linking us to Cuarón's other Oscar winner *Gravity.* He describes DP Lubezki's trademark camera movements and their relationship to background / foreground as "being like two astronauts bound to each other in space … but floating in different directions, seeing different things".

You might argue that it is more a function of Cuarón's standing as a successful auteur that he can command budgets that allow him to 'build' worlds with such huge numbers of extras and props and wide detailed vistas in the background. It's true that the spectacle of Cuarón's universes is normally reserved for superhero, blockbuster or genre films. His films are undoubtedly relatively expensive, but starting with *Y Tu Mamá También*, made with a modest budget of a few million dollars, the director's intent is clear – the background and foreground exchange "weight" and importance throughout the film.

In fact, *Y Tu Mamá También* and *Children of Men* share a scatological scene that provides an illustration of both the technique and continuity in the films. A finger-pulling fart-inducing scene in a car between major characters who are close friends happens early on in both films. The comedy of the scenes, the juvenile silliness of them, is then undercut in both films as the camera floats away and focuses on a more serious part of the world – the fart happening at that very same moment – we then hear / see the desperate plight of the immigrants in *Children of Men* and the death of a construction worker in *Y Tu Mamá También*.

Žižek argues in *The Possibility of Hope* (2007) that this technique of the background is foreground is because

> if you look … too directly at the oppressive social dimension, you don't see it. You can see it in an oblique way only if it remains in the background … The fate of the individual here remains a kind of prism through which you see the background even more sharply.

But in *Roma*, Cleo is seen cleaning shit from the very beginning of the film, and every time one of the family is annoyed about something in their lives they instruct her to clean up, normally the dog shit, that we see in close lurid detail. Scatological jokes are substituted for literal shit, whilst the characters in the background of those films – the immigrants, the workers, are now foregrounded. This is Cleo's story. The Indigenous Mexican, the low-paid maid – a woman clearly marked as 'other' in the household she serves. The technique develops over the films; in *Y Tu Mamá También* a voiceover provides much of the background information; in *Children of Men* it is the roving camera; but in *Roma* it is the background and foreground that merge. The shit, the working people, the ordinary lives are foregrounded and captured in wide screen vistas.

Social realism

In *Roma*, Cuarón wears his heart on his sleeve whilst continuing his radical technique of immersing the viewer in a detailed world. There is, however, a more common term that does fit the film and is regarded by the BFI (Armstrong, 2014) as "typically British".

> Better than any other genre, social realism has shown us to ourselves, pushing the boundaries in the effort to put the experiences of real Britons on the screen, and shaping our ideas of what British cinema can be. While our cinema has experienced all the fluctuations in fortune of Hollywood's first export territory, realism has been Britain's richest gift to world cinema.

Roma may belong to that tradition, even if it was not developed in that milieu, and Cuarón's film-making choices suggest he's likely an Anglophile. All of his films were shot in Mexico or the UK, including the space-bound *Gravity* – and Cuarón lives between London and Italy – *Roma* is a neo–social realist film of sorts. *Roma* does nonetheless expose the class nature of society, the built-in racism and sexism, and allows us to think about this clearly stratified world that is coeval with our own society. The past is the present. The background is the foreground.

In *Roma*, whilst still drawing attention to rich story worlds through some thrilling choreography and set building, Cuarón moves one step past his own style and adds something to this social realism tradition. He goes further than *Children of Men* and literally makes the background, Cleo's life as a maid, the foreground. As political reality in a globalised world, we can argue through social media and 24-hour news, the background truly becomes the foreground. At the same time, the old canons of thought, the old hierarchies are challenged by heterogeneity, by a multitude of voices. Cleo's life – the challenges she faces (mostly male but also along class and race lines as well) are the basis to a film-making that seems to want to give voice to the voiceless, or at worst highlight this life as one equal to any other.

Children of Men and *Y Tu Mamá También* end with loss and the death of a protagonist. In the latter the symbolic mother dies, in the former she survives through Theo's sacrifice. As Anderson (2014) reminds us – "These two films demonstrate that we are as much constituted by the losses we experience as those that we disavow, and the experience of loss can be as much the catalyst of political engagement as of solipsistic withdrawal."

We are reminded that this triptych of globalisation films – set in the present, the recent past and the future, are about mothers, about Gaia even. Mothers and children, the difficulties of pregnancy and mortality pervade the three films. And here I am reminded of Gramsci and Toller (*First Reformed*, Chapter 5), both filled with hope and despair – in Cuarón's films we are asked to hold both simultaneously.

In *Roma*, Cleo is left alone on the roof with all the other maids, as planes (to America) fly over. Half drowned in the ocean, she has admitted her darkest thoughts about the child she lost, and yet she remains 'the mother' to these children, the surrogate mother to Cuarón indeed (represented as he seems to be by the other worldly Pepe – a child who can see the past and the future, who tells stories, a mirror to Cuarón's directing career). As we are invited to share the view of the plane, we call back to the moment Cleo lay here and played dead with Pepe. "I can't talk; I'm dead" he tells her. She copies him and repeats his line back to him, adding that she enjoys being dead. But in *Roma*, Cuarón has finally summoned the unheard to life, the dead have a voice. Here in his masterpiece, he comes full circle and of age, spectacularly utilising a lifetime of craft, honing his unique widescreen view. Long uninterrupted wide takes, deep focus, incredible design, detail and brilliant choreography combine throughout. By Bazin's definition, Cuarón is an impressive auteur with a distinct visual style.

"We are the background" becomes a potential rallying call of hope amongst the hopelessness of the current moment. A cinema of spectacle for a humanism we might call Epic Anamorphic Social Realism.

References

Anderson, J. (2014) 'The Politics of Melancholy in Alfonoso's Cuarón's *Y Tu Mama Tambien, Children of Men* and *The Possibility of Hope*'. *Graduate Student Theses, Dissertations, & Professional Papers*, 4205. https://scholarworks.umt.edu/etd/4205.

Armstrong, R. (2014) *Social Realism*. http://www.screenonline.org.uk/film/id/1037898/.

Brecht, B. (2016) Bertolt Brecht's Dramatic Structure, 25 March. https://news.cah.ucf.edu/news/bertolt-brechts-dramatic-structure/

Brecht, B. (2019) Brecht's Plays. https://literariness.org/2019/05/04/analysis-of-bertolt-brechts-plays/

Breathing Frames (2016) Don't Ignore the Background. https://www.youtube.com/watch?v=fH44hr2Cq2w

Calloway, M. (2014) Isolating Tension: Foreground and Background in Children of Men. https://marielcalloway.com/2014/11/28/isolating-tensions-foreground-background-in-children-of-men/

Coupland, D. (1991) *Generation X*. St Martin's Press.

Cuarón, A. (2007) *The Possibility of Hope (DVD Extra to Children of Men)*.

Fairbairn, W. R. D. (1952) *Psychoanalytic Studies of the Personality*. London: Routledge.

Flisfeder, M. (2017) *Postmodern Theory and Blade Runner*. London: Bloomsbury.

Horvat, S. (2018) '*Children of Men* film talk: Srecko Horvat & Alfonso Cuarón', http://opentranscripts.org/transcript/children-of-men-srecko-horvat-alfonso-Cuarón.

Lowe, J. (2021) 'Los Angeles Goes to War with Itself'. *New York Times*, 13 July.

Thompson / Weiner (2004) 'Mexicans charge former president with 1971 killings'. *New York Times*, 24 July. https://www.nytimes.com/2004/07/24/world/mexicans-charge-a-former-president-with-1971-killings.html

Scott, A. (2020) 'Homelessness in Los Angeles County Rises'. *All Things Considered*, NPR. https://www.npr.org/2020/06/12/875888864/homelessness-in-los-angeles-county-rises-sharply?t=1616695027094

Stahl, T. (2018) 'Georg [György] Lukács', *The Stanford Encyclopedia of Philosophy*, Spring 2018 2018 edition. Edward N. Zalta (ed.). https://plato.stanford.edu/archives/spr2018/entries/Lukács/

Wolmart, G. (2017) 'On Anamorphic Adaptations and the Children of Men'. *International Journal of Žižek Studies*, 11 (2).

5

FIRST REFORMED ((THE OLD GUARD) SCHRADER, 2017)

As Little as Possible; Roads to Freedom

Internal Worlds

Central Self – besieged, Ideal Self – depleted, Antilibidinal Selves – multiplied

The prime candidate for a *Central Self* is doubly compromised. He is Ernst Toller, the (youthful) middle-aged pastor of a beautiful old Dutch Reformed church which has a significant political history of being used to help slaves from the South escape to the North. This church is about to be reconsecrated after 250 years. Almost an historic relic now, it is being preserved by a huge, new, evangelical church, *The Church of Abundant Life*, run by pastor Jeffers, which is substantially funded by a local businessman, Balq, the head of a multinational firm making paper and paper-based goods, who is blocking attempts to reduce environmental pollution.

Toller, a former military pastor, is undergoing a 'dark night of the soul' and has recently started writing a journal signalling his doubts about his faith. We learn that he convinced his son to enlist in the war in Iraq as part of a strong family tradition of service to both the state and religion, and that his son was killed in Iraq aged 19. As a consequence, Toller left the military, and his wife, who strongly opposed her son's decision to enlist, now holds him accountable and has left him.

He is embattled. The death of his son and his wife leaving him have effectively destroyed his *Ideal Self*, and he is left with a punitive *Antilibidinal Self / Internal Saboteur*, the narrator of his journal, alone and in doubt, concerned for his sanity. Physically, he has a worrying persistent cough, stomach pains, vomiting, blood in his urine and stools and he is drinking too much.

DOI: 10.4324/9781003206224-6

Toller has been asked to go to the *Church of Abundant Life* to talk with pastor Jeffers about the up-and-coming reconsecration celebrations. Jeffers, who was instrumental in getting Toller the job, is concerned about Toller's health, spiritually and mentally, and the degree to which the plans are in hand for this prestigious reconsecration, in particular whether the organ has been mended. Later, Toller has coffee with Esther, who leads the choir at the *Church of Abundant Life*, and it is clear that they have had an affair and that she still has feelings for him but that he is no longer interested and finds her interest and concern impinging upon his life. Through her engulfing concern she has become an *Antilibidinal Object* for him.

After the normal low-key service at his church, one of the (sparse) congregation, a young woman, Mary, who is heavily pregnant, approaches Toller and asks him to counsel her husband, Michael, who is worried about the climate crisis to the degree that he wants her to abort the child she is carrying, because he, Michael, cannot think of anything to tell that child when she grows up to a world ravaged by the effects of the climate crisis. Michael is actively imagining the guilt he will feel when his child asks him why he subjected her to this catastrophe, when he knew it would happen.

When Toller talks to Michael, he finds that he has a coherent and convincing view of our apparently inevitable slide into planetary catastrophe and that he wants to avoid subjecting his child to what he sees as unavoidable suffering. Michael represents a possible new *Ideal Self* for the pastor. Although Toller argues against what he sees as the 'dangerous despair' that the young man is falling into. Toller recounts his own experience of losing a child and contrasts his situation of losing his 19-year-old son with Michael's despair at a possible future. Michael asks him how he carried on. Toller responds arguing that courage is the solution for despair, as reason provides no answers. He asks: how can we know what the future will bring? Consequently, we have to choose despite the uncertainty of any particular outcome. He suggests that wisdom is holding two contradictory truths in our mind simultaneously, hope and despair. A life without despair is a life without hope. Holding these two ideas in our head is life itself.

A little later, after asking Toller if he is a drinking man and Toller telling him that it doesn't help, Michael poses the question. "Can God forgive us for what we have done to this world?" To which Toller responds with a question of his own as to who can know the mind of God. All we can do, he says, is choose the righteous life. He says that in his view, belief, forgiveness, grace, covers us all.

Toller is at least partly convinced as to the seriousness and importance of Michael's arguments and commitments and suggests meeting him again to explore things further, as Michael is clearly troubled. Toller, before leaving, asks him sincerely if he is likely to harm himself, which Michael denies.

Before Toller and Michael next meet, Mary contacts Toller and asks him to come to their house, where she shows him a suicide vest that Michael has made and hidden in their garage. Toller takes the suicide vest away to dispose of it and promises not to tell the police.

Having agreed to meet again, Michael texts Toller to reschedule their meeting to a local park. When Toller arrives in the park, he finds that Michael has killed himself with a shotgun. This represents another blow to Toller's already weakened *Ideal* and *Central Selves.*

Later, while Toller is at the couple's house comforting Mary, he finds Michael's 'Last Will and Testament' in an envelope addressed to him. Toller carries out the young man's instructions for a memorial ceremony and the disposal of his ashes in a derelict and polluted area of the city, supposedly cleaned up by Balq's firm. Michael has requested a small choir from the *Church of Abundant Life* to sing a Neil Young song, 'Who's gonna stand up and save the earth?', to the small gathering of friends and family, before Mary spreads Michael's ashes at the site.

Toller, shaken by the young man's death, uses Michael's collection of data on the climate crisis to begin to look more critically at the problem, and the part played by big business in climate crisis denial. In particular, the political part played by the local businessman in preventing effective measures to help stem the climate catastrophe.

At a meeting between Toller, Balq and Jeffers to discuss the forthcoming 250th anniversary of Toller's church, and its reconsecration, Balq starts an argument accusing Toller of meddling in things he doesn't understand and being inappropriately political, citing a web-based report of the recent memorial service for Michael. They argue, and Toller disagrees with Balq over the climate crisis and cites the overwhelming scientific consensus. During the argument Toller asks Balq the question he was asked by Michael: "Can God forgive us?" Balq treats the question with contempt, and when he finds out that Toller had counselled Michael before he killed himself, he is even more contemptuous of Toller's right to say anything.

Toller decides to consult a doctor over his health issues. He has blood in his urine and stools, he has night cramps and fits of vomiting, all of which suggest something like cancer of the stomach or bowel. The doctor offers him advice on his diet, and drinking, and books him in to have an endoscopic investigation of his stomach and gut.

Mary asks Toller to help her clear some of Michael's clothes and other things related to the climate crisis, and Toller looks again at the climate crisis evidence in more depth and at a film of a man killing himself using a suicide vest.

As the reconsecration celebration approaches, Jeffers suggests that Toller not run the celebration, which Toller resists strongly, agreeing to go into rehab immediately after the reconsecration.

One night, Mary visits Toller, clearly disturbed, and he asks her how she calmed herself when this happened previously. She tells him that Michael was really strong, he listened, he was kind. She tells him that they used to do this thing called the Magical Mystery Tour. They would share a joint, lay on top of each other fully clothed, and try to get as much body-to-body contact as possible. With arms outstretched looking straight into each other's eyes moving them in unison right, left, right, left, as they breathed in rhythm.

Toller asks Mary if she wants them to do this. Mary agrees after a brief hesitation. Soon after her lying on top of him, they are shown floating up into the air together and out into space across snow-covered mountains, above valleys and oceans, over forests. Then the flight takes a darker path, over derelict cars, scrapyards full of tyres, smoking factories, ruined landscapes, rubbish, fires, representing the process of their shared imagination moving from a benign state to a horrifying one. This intimacy and that ecstatic / transcendent experience signalling some deeply shared, if disturbing, experience.

Toller remains clearly conflicted, however. We see him trying on the suicide vest and preparing it for use by mending it. We see him talking to Mary about the anticipated birth of her child, and planning to visit her when she is living with her sister in Buffalo. She asks about the reconsecration of the church and says that she will be there for him as he has been there for her. He puts her off and insists that she shouldn't go to the reconsecration, which confirms what we already suspected, that he is going to use the suicide vest at the reconsecration ceremony himself.

Later, Toller cleans the grounds of the church, taking some barbed wire off the low fences, and then, later, visits Balq's factory where a guide tells a party of tourists about the good, green, work the factory and the industry are doing.

As the reconsecration ceremony gets underway, Toller puts on the suicide vest and arms it. As the people wait for him to start the ceremony, he sees Mary entering the church and becomes distraught. He cannot kill himself if it will possibly kill her and her unborn baby too. He removes the suicide vest and wraps himself in the barbed wire he has retrieved from the garden, causing him to bleed with the sort of scourge marks a tormented Christ figure might have. Meanwhile Jeffers has got tired of waiting with his important guests and goes looking for Toller; the Governor and Balq are also getting impatient in the front pews and Jeffers, unable to find Toller, gets the choir mistress, Esther, to start the proceedings by singing the hymn "Leaning on the everlasting arms".

Toller in a white robe, blood stained from his many scourging wounds seeping through it, pours himself a glass of *Drano* in order to finish himself off, when Mary appears at the door and calls out his first name, "Ernst!" He rushes into her arms, and they are united in a loving embrace. She and her developing baby have become his *Ideal* and *Libidinal* others supporting his *Central Self* and offering him a way back towards some degree of wholeness and a new life with a renewed *Ideal Self*, based on the redemptive power of a pregnant woman.

This redemptive figure of the pregnant Mary, which has obvious Catholic overtones, offers new possibilities for a way forward and some hope for the near psychotic Toller, beset on all sides by the threat of fragmentation and illusory martyrdom, to make something like a proper *restitution* and begin to heal. Or is it, as Schrader seems to indicate in some of his interviews, a miracle?

Guilt and the moral defence

In a 2018 interview Schrader is characterised as being "known for his intense style of cinema, fuelled by certain thematic preoccupations that come straight out of his strict religious upbringing—the paralyzing power of guilt, the self-destructive impulse, the possibility of redemption" (Cortellessa, 2018). In Chapter III section 6 entitled 'Guilt as a Defence Against the Release of Bad Objects' (Fairbairn, 1952) Fairbairn discusses the 'Moral Defence'.

> The essential feature, and indeed the essential aim, of this defence is the conversion of an original situation in which the child is surrounded by bad objects into a new situation in which his objects are good and he himself is bad. The moral situation which results belongs, of course, to a higher level of mental development than the original situation; and this level is characteristically a 'civilized' level. It is the level at which the super-ego operates, and to which the interplay between the ego and the super-ego belongs. It is the level at which analytical interpretations in terms of guilt and the Oedipus situation are alone applicable; and it would appear to be the level at which psychotherapy is often rather exclusively conducted.
>
> *(pp. 68–70)*

However, for Fairbairn, the super-ego is a complex structure made up of the punitive antilibidinal self and the positive ego-ideal / ideal-object. "What Freud described as the 'superego' is really a complex structure comprising (a) the ideal object or ego-ideal, (b) the antilibidinal ego, and (c) the rejecting (or antilibidinal) object" (Fairbairn, 1963, pp. 224–225). Fairbairn's subsequent thoughts about some difficulties of analysis may help us to make sense of Michael's tragic suicide.

> An analysis conducted too exclusively at the guilt or super-ego level may, however, easily have the effect of producing a negative therapeutic reaction; for the removal of a patient's defence of guilt may be accompanied by a compensatory access of repression which renders the resistance impenetrable. There is now little doubt in my mind that … the deepest source of resistance is fear of the release of bad objects from the unconscious; for, when such bad objects are released, the world around the patient becomes peopled with devils which are too terrifying for him to face … it is only when the internalized bad objects are released from the

> unconscious that there is any hope of their cathexis being dissolved. The bad objects can only be safely released, however, if the analyst has become established as a sufficiently good object for the patient. Otherwise, the resulting insecurity may prove insupportable. Given a satisfactory transference situation, a therapeutically optimal release of bad objects can, in my opinion, only be promoted if caution is exercised over interpretations at the guilt or super-ego level. Whilst such interpretations may relieve guilt, they may actually have the effect of intensifying the repression of internalized bad objects and thus leaving the cathexis of these objects unresolved. It is to the realm of these bad objects, I feel convinced, rather than to the realm of the super-ego that the ultimate origin of all psychopathological developments is to be traced; for it may be said of all psychoneurotic and psychotic patients that, if a True Mass is being celebrated in the chancel, a Black Mass is being celebrated in the crypt. It becomes evident, accordingly, that the psychotherapist is the true successor to the exorcist, and that he is concerned, not only with 'the forgiveness of sins', but also with 'the casting out of devils'.
>
> *(Fairbairn, 1963, p. 70)*

The problem being that Toller, during his brief counselling of Michael, has been unable to achieve either.

Thomas Merton and the dark night of the soul

Toller reads Thomas Merton on and off throughout the film, and the following quote from Merton may resonate with Toller's feelings as he is writing his journal. I would argue that it can be seen as an account of what it might be like to approach *Mature Dependence* as Fairbairn saw it.

> During the 'dark night' of the feelings and senses, anxiety is felt in prayer, often acutely. This is necessary, because this spiritual night marks the transfer of the full, free control of our inner life into the hands of a superior power. And this too means that the time of darkness is, in reality, a time of hazard and of difficult options. We begin to go out of ourselves: that is to say, we are drawn out from behind our habitual and conscious defences. These defences are also limitations, which we must abandon if we are to grow. But at the same time, they are, in their own way, a protection against the unconscious forces that are too great for us to face naked and without protection … If we set out into this darkness, we have to meet these inexorable forces. We will have to face fears and doubts. We will have to call into question the whole structure of our spiritual life. We will have to make a new evaluation of our motives for belief, for love, for self-commitment to the invisible God. And at this moment, precisely, all spiritual light is darkened, all values lose their

> shape and reality, and we remain, so to speak, suspended in the void … The most crucial aspect of this experience is precisely the temptation to doubt God himself. We must not minimize the fact that this is a genuine risk. For here we are advancing beyond the stage where God made himself accessible to our mind in simple and primitive images. We are entering the night in which he is present without any image, invisible, inscrutable, and beyond any satisfactory mental representation … At such a time as this, one who is not seriously grounded in genuine theological faith may lose everything he ever had. His prayer may become an obscure and hateful struggle to preserve the images and trappings which covered his own interior emptiness. Either he will have to face the truth of his emptiness or else he will beat a retreat into the realm of images and analogies which no longer serve for a mature spiritual life. He may not be able to face the terrible experience of being apparently without faith in order to really grow in faith. For it is this testing, this fire of purgation, that burns out the human and accidental elements of faith in order to liberate the deep spiritual power in the centre of our being. This gift of God is, of itself, unattainable, but is given to us moment by moment, beyond our comprehension, by his inscrutable mercy.
>
> *(Thomas Merton, 2005, pp. 77–78)*

External Worlds

> It's freezing in NYC. Where the hell is global warming?
>
> *(Donald Trump, Tweet, Dec 2017)*

The old new wave

Paul Schrader's *First Reformed* (2017) is a bleak but brilliant film of transcendence, about a crisis of faith and a crisis of climate. It is one of three films influenced by Scorsese and Schrader's *Taxi Driver* that are considered in this book; *Joker* and *You Were Never Really Here* being the other two.

First Reformed questions why, as a species, we still fiddle while Rome burns. Where the hell are we with the most pressing question of the day and what are we to do? It's a question Schrader takes seriously, as opposed to the mocking tones of his erstwhile president. Significantly, one of Trump's first acts was to remove the US from the Paris Climate Treaty, on the basis that it would undermine the American economy. Trump is an avowed climate change sceptic. In contrast, Schrader addresses the urgent, violent question of climate change in the moment, and puts his voice firmly on the side of radicalism.

Schrader was a part of the 1970s American new wave generation of film school–educated movie brats. During that decade, a group of directors that knew each other well – Coppola, Scorsese and De Palma amongst their number, created lasting classics like *Mean Streets, Nashville, The Godfather,*

The Conversation, Chinatown, Apocalypse Now and the aforementioned *Taxi Driver*. At the same time, two others from the group also paved the way for the modern event movie: Steven Spielberg and George Lucas making *Jaws, Star Wars, ET* and *Raiders of the Lost Ark* in the space of just five years and revolutionising cinema production up until the present day. The blockbuster event movie they helped create now dominates studio production, including the comic book universes that Scorsese recently railed against (see Chapter 7, *Joker*). Much of this period and its films (including *Taxi Driver*) are documented entertainingly in Peter Biskind's *Easy Riders, Raging Bulls* (1999) and analysed critically in Kolker's *A Cinema of Loneliness* (2011).

If *Taxi Driver* looks at "God's lonely man" (Wolfe, 1930) and establishes a new version of the cinema of the outsider, *First Reformed* is its eco-sequel. Schrader's films have always been deeply personal, and at the same time heavily influenced by Bresson – repeating the same themes of alienation, loneliness, isolation – and transcendence too. As mentioned, he has laid out his process, both as a writer, in his lectures (Schrader, 2018b), and, as outlined in his now reissued book, his influences (Schrader, 2018a).

First Reformed shares many themes and tropes with *Taxi Driver*. Travis and Toller both speak their increasingly dark diaries, and are filled with moral rage, loneliness, self-destructiveness and the despising of everyone including oneself. Coming towards the end of Schrader's career, *First Reformed* seems to bookend with *Taxi Driver*, not only thematically and tonally but also in terms of its strong critical reception, nominated as it was for an Academy Award for Original Screenplay.

Metaphor, problem and The Presentation of Self in Everyday Life

> Can God forgive us for what we've done to this world?
>
> *(Reverend Ernst Toller,* First Reformed*)*

In his BAFTA lectures (2018b) Schrader talks of finding the metaphor and the problem in films like *Taxi Driver, American Gigolo, Raging Bull* and *First Reformed*:

> I did a film about loneliness … out of a dark period of wandering and being ungrounded, and I was sort of living in my car and had a pain in my stomach and went to the hospital and had a bleeding ulcer at the age of twenty-five, because I was just drinking and driving. And in the hospital, I got this image of a taxicab. It came to me, this yellow, rectangular coffin, a metal coffin floating through the open sewers of a metropolis, and inside that coffin is trapped a young man. And it looks like he's surrounded by life but he's absolutely alone. The power of that metaphor just overwhelmed me.

He goes on to explain how both his idea of metaphor and of problem are related:

> Now what is a metaphor? A metaphor is the stand-in, it is not the problem itself. So, the metaphor for a lonely boy is not a lonely boy, a metaphor for an unattractive girl is not an unattractive girl. It's something like the metaphor, and like the problem, but not the problem itself. It's like two wires, you have the problem and the metaphor; and they have to get close enough for a spark to jump across. And if they're too far apart there'll be no spark and if they're on top of each other there'll be no spark … A metaphor can sometimes be an occupation – a taxi driver … and one of the things I'd been talking with my psychiatrist about was the inability to express love and now I'm teaching … and I happened to say to the class, 'what occupation does this person have? Are they a factory worker? Bookkeeper? Doctor? Gigolo? Lawyer?' And boom. And as soon as I said the word 'gigolo' it was boom; you've got your metaphor. That's the metaphor you've been looking for, for the inability to express love. Now I had a problem, now I had a metaphor; I was on my way.

Schrader refers to looking for the right character, the right metaphor and the right problem when writing a film. He goes beyond the structural prescriptions of Syd Field et al., to look at what his prospective film is about and how characters can embody that. In *First Reformed*, he takes his Calvinist obsessions, his cinematic influences, his anxieties about ageing and a dying planet and looks not only at a man who has cut himself off from the world in Toller, but at a man who is forced, by his relationship with two of his dwindling congregation, to re-engage with the world in a shocking and meaningful way. While many films have dealt with the future consequences of the Anthropocene, Schrader tackles not only the existential questions: *who am I and why am I?* but also a much larger existential question: *will my species survive?* and, as a Christian: *will God forgive us for destroying nature?* And most crucially, following on from this and making the theological political: *what would God have me do?*

Toller, the priest of the First Reformed church, engages with one of his flock, Michael, at the behest of the man's wife, Mary. A climate activist, Michael, who has already been imprisoned for his beliefs, discusses his future child with Toller and asks him how he can, in good conscience, bring a child into the world knowing that the planet is already dying. In an early scene at his house, Michael presents a compelling argument for man's imminent demise and the nonchalance of the world to climate change and in particular big business's role in obfuscation, deliberately hiding the true state of things to preserve their profits. He even presents the shocking but barely talked about reality that climate activists are regularly killed for their beliefs (Butt et al., 2019).

Toller encourages Michael to show wisdom by holding despair and hope in the same thought, but Michael, having denied that he is thinking of harming himself to Toller, kills himself a few days later. Toller has already lost a son to the Iraq War. He has a long history of military service in his family, but he is now disillusioned. As Toller confesses, he talked his son into a war with no moral justification and his son was killed, so Toller left the military. Toller appears to us from the outset already a beaten man – his son dead, his wife having left him, it seems his failure to stop Michael's suicide opens the path to radicalism for himself. This is in stark contrast to Glass in *The Revenant*, who is able to use his dead son and wife as internal resources for his own persistence and courage, whereas Toller is heading towards self-immolation.

On the one hand, Toller presents to the world as a man of the cloth, deeply religious, thoughtful, leading his small congregation and taking tours for schools. He is kind to schoolchildren, listens to Michael, offers him hope and prays with his bereaved wife, the aptly named Mary. The diary that he reads, (and that we hear in voiceover), and the way it contradicts Toller's daily work and private life, reveals the huge fissures in his world. He professes not to drink, or to drink only wine, and yet we often see him pour whiskey as he writes, and his bin is full of empties. The chilling mix that he pours of Pepto-Bismol and whiskey brilliantly mirrors the haunting images of oil slicks and pollution throughout the film. It also foreshadows the thick bleach he pours to kill himself at the end. Toller is in extreme pain, both physical – bleeding, vomiting, coughing – and existential – raging, screaming, calling out to God for help – but he hides this as best he can from his church, the congregation, his ex-lover, the caretaker and his boss, the head of the super Church of Abundant Life. At various times we see Toller's inner life, what Goffman called "the backstage". He feels he cannot speak, and when he does, he reveals too much. Occasionally he betrays this turmoil – most particularly at a lunch date with his church leader and arch polluter Balq to prepare the way for the 250th anniversary of the church.

His presentation of self is important. He is a priest after all. A man of God. As Goffman (1959) says in the remarkably prescient "Presentation of Self in Everyday Life":

> … and to the degree that the individual maintains a show before others that he himself does not believe, he can come to experience a special kind of alienation from self and a special kind of wariness of others.

Toller's encounter with Michael, his growing intimacy with Mary and his confrontation with Balq accelerate this ongoing crisis. Michael chooses Toller to fulfil the wishes of his will, including a macabre funeral in front of a polluted stretch of a local waterway. It is like a scene from Tarkovsky's *Stalker* – here we see parts of Toller's local neighbourhood are already scorched and destroyed. Michael is buried in front of his predicted fear of the future world. These images are added to and expanded when we magically pass from an image of Toller and Mary lying on his bare living room floor together into a "metaphysical trip". Man's destruction of God's creation is laid bare in this trip into nature's beauty, mountain tops and forests through to abandoned tyres and rotting terrain. As Schrader says in *Transcendental Style*, "the supernatural in film is only the real rendered more precise. Real things seen close up" (Schrader, 2018b, p. 82).

It is worth noting the formal aspects of Schrader's work in *First Reformed* here. He shoots in a tight 4:3 aspect ratio, and the camera rarely moves for the entire first half of the film. Similarly, an ominous tonal music is a late arrival in the, until now, scoreless film, coming as it does over the metaphysical union of Mary and Toller. This same sequence and the climactic embrace between Mary and Toller are two of the few moments when the camera moves, in a similar circular fashion around the protagonists. The absence of movement before this moment accentuates the unbearable tension further. This style underlines Toller's pain, his austere way of living, his self-flagellation – the prison of the frame being the prison of his own tortured mind. Everything is stripped back to its essentials, laid bare. The economy in Schrader's script and direction is impressive. No shot goes wasted, no scene is extraneous to the theme, the metaphor, the questions. The script's economy is exemplary, the complete opposite to the comic book movie (as discussed in Chapter 7, *Joker*). In *First Reformed*, the spectacle is spare but effective. The film comes to life through the characters, their actions, the dialogue and themes explored in great detail and to powerful dramatic effect. As Schrader says, quoting Bresson, "A film is not a spectacle, it is in the first place a Style" (Schrader, 2018b, p. 60).

First Reformed *and* Diary of a Country Priest *by Robert Bresson*

As Schrader notes, there are some striking parallels between *First Reformed* and the *Diary of a Country Priest* by Robert Bresson, in terms of the main narrative and down to some of the details of the ways in which the journal is being written – apologies, partial retractions, pages torn out and destroyed. That Schrader is influenced by Bresson's film is clear from his own film and his book, *Transcendental Style in Cinema* (2018b).

The country priest has stomach problems and difficulties eating, as does Toller. He is writing a journal about the difficulties of his ministry and the local people, he is in conflict with the local 'bigwigs' and consults a fellow priest about his problems, as does Toller. In Bresson's film the country priest does manage to help the Count's wife to come to terms with her son's tragic death and regain some peace, another parallel to Toller, who has sent his son to be killed in the war in Iraq, about which he still feels guilty. The country priest is also at loggerheads with the Count, as Toller is with the climate change–denying big businessman Balq.

There is some ambivalence in the relationships between the country priest and the Count's daughter Chantal, and with a girl in his catechism class,

Seraphita. These are at one and the same time agonistic and libidinal, whereas Toller's relationship with Mary is increasingly tender and libidinal.

There is a suicide in both films, for example, when Dr Delbende, who the country priest has consulted, kills himself with a shotgun, in much the same way that Matthew did whilst consulting Toller. Suicide is also discussed with the Countess and with one of the local priests, who is quite happy to bury the doctor, accepting the story that he has had a shooting accident without inspecting the possibility of suicide seriously, which would prevent him from giving him a Catholic burial.

Perhaps the major difference between the two films is the way the films end. In one the country priest succumbs to his stomach cancer and dies painfully, in the other the stomach cancer, if that is what it is, gets treated, and despite his strong urges to martyr himself Toller is rescued by the love of a good woman, who in herself represents the archetype of the Roman Catholic Church and the Virgin Mary, complete with the unborn child.

At the end of Bresson's film, the country priest, desperately ill with stomach cancer, is staying with a friend he originally met in the seminary, who is also ill; when they discuss breaking their vows and leaving the church, his friend says that he would only do this on intellectual grounds, but the country priest says he would only do it for the love of a woman, which is what, you might argue, happens in *First Reformed.*

An exceptional end of the world

> "I want you to act as if the house is on fire, because it is."
>
> *(Thunberg, 2019)*

The rise of the apocalypse movie (from *Planet of the Apes* through to *World War Z, I am Legend, A Quiet Place, The Road* and even including *Avengers Endgame*) shows us the end of the world in its various possible forms. Then there is a separate pantheon that includes films such as *Mad Max: Fury Road* and *The Day After Tomorrow* that have ecological strands to their apocalyptic future as opposed to alien invasion, rise of the zombies, death by meteor, death by disease and nuclear war. A third strand, including films like *Elysium* and *Blade Runner*, show a world where life on Earth is a poor relation to off-world colonies, whilst a fourth, which includes films such as *Interstellar* and *The Midnight Sky*, feature ecological disaster in the near future but offer up some individual hope for survival through the power of love.

Nolan's *Interstellar* examines the consequences and responses to an unfolding or already happening ecological disaster. Like all of these films, the end of the world or at least our current civilisation has already happened. *Elysium* and *Blade Runner* similarly look at an Earth that is almost uninhabitable. At best a "Favelerisation" of the planet. A planet of slums where the ruling class have all escaped off-world thanks to androids and currently impossible technologies. What Bruce Sterling called "Favela Chic" (2009), the idea that people could be plugged into the internet, social media and all the attenuated benefits of online life but at the same time work in what he described at the time as a 'McJob' with low wages and poor conditions, is represented as parable in these films.

But the reality is even worse. I spent a jetlagged week in Santa Barbara for the film festival in 2019. Waking at 5 a.m. every day, I'd go to one of three Starbucks to catch up with the UK online and grab coffee. The other early morning occupants were exclusively the homeless of the town. The most shocking thing, however, was that most had smart phones or tablets that they used to access the digital world all day, but no real access to basic amenities including healthcare and housing. I lived in Downtown LA as a homeless person in 2007 for the documentary film *Skid Row* (2007), and this brief encounter with the homeless American life that blights at least half a million people was traumatic and brutal. Chris Arnade's (2019) work in *The Guardian* and his book *Dignity* (2019) tells the full and desperately sad story of these blighted lives, echoing as it does George Packer's *The Unwinding: Thirty Years of American Decline* (2013) and John Dos Passos's *U.S.A.* trilogy (1930–36). Post-Covid, the combined homeless and prison population of the US stands at 1 per cent of the population – unprecedented among the rich G7 nations.

Perhaps less a case of William Gibson's aphoristic "the future is here, it's just not evenly distributed" than "the future is everywhere but the basics of income, housing and health care have been obliterated".

> Fredric Jameson suggests that the predominance of dystopic visions in contemporary science fiction signals the general loss of our ability even to conceive of, much less struggle to enact, a utopian social vision, trapped as we are within both an imperialist nation in decline and the overheated 'perpetual present' of postmodernist culture.
>
> *(Pfeil, 1993 p. 244)*

If the present was overheated pre-social media, pre iPhone, then it's well above Paris Accord levels in 2021. These films allow us to ignore the present moment, the fact that "our house is on fire".

Our present moment is now our science fiction, complicated, alien, slippery, as Rothman (2019) puts it, "Midway through his career the inventor of cyberspace turned his attention to a strange new world – 'the present'". Gibson himself, in *Pattern Recognition* (2003), talks about the problem of now, the present moment, today:

> We have no future … For us, of course, things can change so abruptly, so violently, so profoundly, that futures like our grandparents' have

> insufficient "now" to stand on. We have no futures because our present is too volatile …. We have only risk management. The spinning of the given moment's scenarios.

Gibson and Schrader take the road less travelled, but most films offer up yet to be invented technology or pure love or miracles to solve ecological problems of planetary existence. *Interstellar* offers up such a vision. These are wish-fulfilment dreams at best, irresponsible myths at worst. They fit with the worldview of billionaire influencer Elon Musk and his Space X Mars colonisation programme. As Lizzie O'Shea (2019, p. 109) notes after watching Werner Herzog's *Lo and Behold: Reveries of the Connected World*:

> Herzog interviews Musk about his plan to settle humans on Mars; Musk claims it is "in case something goes wrong" with Earth. In response the astronomer Lucianne Walkowicz points out … that the "focus on making Mars habitable distracts us from the fact that we are currently making Earth uninhabitable" …. Musk's plan is to buy and exploit his way out of a dysfunctional society with his own self-designed utopia.

Returning to making the theological political – *what would God have me do?* More urgently and specifically: *what can we do to avert this disaster*? Films like *Interstellar* and *The Midnight Sky* posit a future where disaster is inevitable. There is literally nothing that can be done. Do they then have the opposite effect to that intended, dissolving into dangerous films of apathy and hopelessness, rather than a present call to arms? The end of the world in all its technicolour glory as Thanatosis, as perverse pleasure. Faced with ecological disaster, America, arch polluter, has few answers other than denial or projection into an unknown future.

As Fisher (2009) puts it, when discussing Pixar's *Wall-E*,

> The film shows an earth so despoiled that human beings are no longer capable of inhabiting it. We're left in no doubt that consumer capitalism and corporations – or rather one mega-corporation, *Buy n Large* – is responsible for this depredation; and when we eventually see the human beings in offworld exile, they are infantile and obese, interacting via screen interfaces, carried around in large motorized chairs, and supping indeterminate slop from cups. This kind of irony feeds rather than challenges capitalist realism. A film like Wall-E exemplifies what Robert Pfaller has called 'interpassivity': the film performs our anti-capitalism for us, allowing us to continue to consume with impunity … capitalism can proceed perfectly well, in some ways better.

A Transformation

> There must be at a certain moment, be a transformation; if not, there is no art.
> *(Schrader, 2018a, p. 82)*

Towards the end of *First Reformed*, as it becomes clear that Toller is set upon a radical and violent path to speak up for the planet, Toller copies quotations from the Bible (including *Revelations*) into his diary.

> Be strong in the Lord and his mighty power. Put on the full armour of God. So that you can take your stand against the devil's schemes. For our struggle is not against flesh and blood, but against the rulers, against the authorities, against the powers of this dark world.
> *(Ephesians 6:10)*

There is no ambiguity here. His anger, like Michael's, is aimed firmly at the corporate polluters who also fund his church – most particularly Ed Balq. He is caught in the nexus of capitalist relations. Even in his small church, where he has sought refuge from the world, his family history in the military, his grief, he is faced with the bitter irony that he is funded by capitalism.

The history of the undermining of the green movement is part of the neoliberal project, as explained by Philip Mirowski (2013):

> The promotion of denialism buys time for the other two options; the financialization of carbon credits gets all the attention in the medium term, while appeals to geoengineering incubate in the wings as a techno-utopian deus ex machina to swoop down when the other options fail. At each step along the way, the neoliberals guarantee their core tenet remains in force: the market will arbitrate any and all responses to biosphere degradation, because it knows more than any of us about nature and society.

As Mirowski goes onto say in a later essay, 'Hell Is Truth Seen Too Late' (2019), neoliberalism aims to hide itself in plain sight and convince us it doesn't exist (much like Keyser Soze in *The Usual Suspects* or Fisher's work in *Capitalist Realism*). This is encapsulated during a scene at the midpoint of the film. The midpoint of a film is often a place where the thesis is discussed and a turning point in the protagonist's trajectory occurs. For Toller, meeting Ed Balq, the CEO of a polluting company, personifies the problem that Michael and now in turn, Toller, can clearly see.

Balq tells Toller his service for Michael's funeral at a toxic waste site was a "political act". Toller, silent for a while, asks Balq, "Will God forgive us for what we are doing to his creation?" echoing Michael's words. "There's been a lot of loose talk about environmental change … It's a complicated subject", Balq continues. "Not really", Toller retorts. "I mean, who profits?" Balq cuts the conversation short by cruelly reminding Toller that after he had counselled Michael, he shot himself. Balq clearly stands in here for the climate deniers – "the powers of this dark world".

As Toller reminds himself in voiceover, "Why couldn't I just keep silent?" But he doesn't, and he won't. His voice and his violence, the backstage of his life as a priest for a super church financially associated with a serial mass polluter, inevitably come boiling up to the surface in a heady, bloody denouement.

The Futility of Good Intentions

For Kolker (2011, p. 54) the 1970s films of Penn and Coppola (notably *The Conversation* and *Night Moves*) mark the "end of the modernist movement in American Cinema … its bleakness and desolation … its conviction that failure and isolation are the only ends available to a male character". Similarly, in his searing study of *Chinatown* (1974) and the four men involved – producer Robert Evans, star Jack Nicholson, writer Robert Towne and director Roman Polanski, Sam Wasson describes the period (and specifically 1974) as representing

> the final flowering of a film garden passionately tended by liberated studio executives and an unspoken agreement between audiences and filmmakers. As Towne had once observed, the American films of World War II benefited from shared beliefs; now, "there was a common assumption that something was wrong," he said, "in the wake of Vietnam and Watergate and assassinations and riots" that gave rise to "a hunger on both sides for something new" and produced a Hollywood year as powerful as 1974. But the poison was in the perfume: These films, Towne said, "did their jobs too well. There was"—presently—"nothing left to expose. There were other films … *Network, Nashville, Taxi Driver* and *The Deer Hunter*, that would hold up a black mirror to fallen America, but the wreckage of Chinatown, transmitted metaphorically, transcends its story and characters. *Chinatown* is a condition. The condition is the terrible awareness of one's helplessness, what Towne had always called "the futility of good intentions."
>
> *(Wasson, 2020, p. 271)*

That this period of American cinema from *Bonnie and Clyde* (and the 1968 backdrop of Tarantino's *Once Upon a Time in Hollywood*) through to *Raging Bull* coincides with failure in Vietnam, Watergate, the oil crisis, high inflation, the Iran hostage crisis and the eventual election of actor turned Monetarist consiglieri Reagan should not surprise us. Jameson, Fisher, Harvey, Curtis and others have identified this period as the transition from a revolutionary moment to a decade of retreat and defeat (the 1980s) – the rise of neoliberalism and the rapid acceleration of globalisation. Films like the ones mentioned above and *The Parallax View, Klute*, reminded us of this futility and Schrader clearly returns to this feeling, the blind alleys of white male anger and impotence in *First Reformed.* It is significant that *Chinatown* ends with the Gittes' muttered line "As little as possible", a mantra that inaction is the only sane action in a world ruled by big business interests.

At the same time, MeToo and Time's Up have, in the last five years, successfully challenged the role of the American White Man in Hollywood and the world. The Age of Aquarius may have been successfully incorporated into the system and commodified effectively, but the upside of the end of modernism and the nascent neoliberal nexus was the proliferation of other points of view beyond the white man. Whilst patriarchal capitalism reasserted itself on one level over America, sometime soon after the Manson murders (see Chapter 11) voices seldom heard developed in film and broke through sporadically, until the recent significant moment for diverse voices. This book is partly about those new voices but also a brief examination of the male-dominated old guards – the New American Cinema of the 1970s and the burgeoning indie world that directors like Soderbergh, the Coens and Jarmusch helped create and Harvey Weinstein grew and exploited.

End of Days for a Generation

Quentin Tarantino, as we shall see, mourns his own demise in *Once Upon a Time in Hollywood* by romanticising the good old days of the 1960s in much the same way as Trump wants to 'Make America Great Again' by reifying some imaginary ideal of the pre–civil rights 1950s.

Schrader and Scorsese, two directors who span this entire period whilst remaining avowedly modernist, take different, more regretful approaches to their own oeuvre in their latest works. *First Reformed* and *The Irishman* offer some small hope of looking back by two such men, not in anger, but by questioning the very life you led, the art you made. They are films full of regret. Films that recognise their generations failings, their own sins. *First Reformed* sees some transcendental redemption through love, or at least the fever dream of it.

In *The Irishman*, Scorsese, having shown a lifetime of men killing, raping and destroying lives, presents a more melancholic viewpoint of the real consequences of that lifestyle and the hopelessness of that personality. *The Irishman* offers up a long retirement for its protagonist, a brutal hitman Frank, to reflect at leisure upon his sins. The final brooding act of the film is depressing and contrary to Scorsese's earlier films of violent men – *Taxi Driver, Raging Bull, Goodfellas, Casino.* In the final scene, Frank has little to say, and what he does finally say is revelatory. "What kind of guy makes a call like that?" is one of the few clues to the back door into Frank's inner life. The "guy" in question refers directly to himself, specifically to his ability to kill and then lie to the widow of the deceased associate he murdered. It is clear that Frank has spent a long time sitting in the half-light to think on this, and when he asks the priest to leave the door to his care room half open, it feels like a muted cry for redemption that will never come.

Is it a coincidence that at this time of their lives, in their mid-70s, long-time partners Scorsese and Schrader both turn to films about the sins of the past? Scorsese offers up hopelessness, impotency and regret whilst Schrader offers up a call to activism and real discernment about the state of the planet, even if his ending holds up the eternal hope of a woman's love – real or imagined.

Joe Biden and Martin Scorsese were both born in 1942. Donald Trump and Paul Schrader were both born in 1946. They are men of a certain generation. One president is for a liberal tweak of the neoliberal status quo, the other for breaking the system, but these two old directors seem less concerned with 'Making America Great Again' and more with making amends, finding some peace in a way that challenges the mistakes of their own generation. They don't offer up solutions but both seem prepared to stare into the abyss and reflect on how it might be different.

Schrader has few answers, but he appears to be still asking the right questions.

Astra Taylor, an Occupy activist and documentary filmmaker (whose work includes Žižek!), writes in her book *Democracy May Not Exist* (2019, p. 307) about the contradictions of the present moment: "While imprisoned by fascists in 1929 Antonio Gramsci wrote to his brother … 'I'm a pessimist because of intelligence … and an optimist because of will'". Leading on from this, she inverts the idea, and by reference to the past, to the history of struggle, concludes, "The established order is so big and powerful, and a single individual so vulnerable and small. But when I engage my intellect, something approaching optimism is possible. The past is proof it can be done" (2019, p. 308). Good films make us think, and husband the will to act rather than pacify our fears.

Hope and despair. Toller echoes this throughout. In *First Reformed*, Schrader's nods to the past (the Iraq War, the Underground Railroad, the teachings of Christ as radical), his survey of the present through the priest's struggle, his belief in the transcendence of love, these offer up something much more than the ubiquitous hero films of technically well imagined futures of apocalypse and environmental collapse. But he has no clear answer. Hopefully, the road to human survival, freedom even, can be enunciated and created by the next generation as this Old Guard gives way.

References

Arnade, C. (2019) 'Our forgotten towns: struggle, resilience, love and respect in "back-row America"'. *The Guardian*. https://www.theguardian.com/us-news/2019/jun/05/america-dignity-chris-arnade-book-extract-poverty

Biskind, P. (1999) *Easy Riders, Raging Bulls*. London: Bloomsbury.

Butt, N., Lambrick, F., Menton, M. et al. (2019) 'The supply chain of violence'. *Nat Sustain* 2: 742–747. https://doi.org/10.1038/s41893-019-0349-4.

Cortellessa, E. (2018) Interview with Schrader. https://slate.com/culture/2018/06/first-reformeds-ending-paul-schrader-explains-why-its-designed-to-be-ambiguous.html.

Fairbairn W. R. D. (1952) *Psychoanalytic Studies of the Personality*. London: RKP.

Fairbairn, W. R. D. (1963) 'Synopsis of an Object-Relations Theory of the Personality'. *International Journal of Psycho-Analysis*, 44: 224–225.

Kolker (2011) *A Cinema of Loneliness*, 4th edition. Oxford University Press.

Fisher, M. (2009) *Capitalist Realism: Is There No Alternative?* London: Zero Books.

Gibson, W. (2003) *Pattern Recognition*. London: Penguin.

Goffman, E. (1959) *The Presentation of Self in Everyday Life*. Scotland: Doubleday.

Merton, T. (2005) *Contemplative Prayer*. Darton, Longman & Todd Ltd.

Mirowski, P. (2013) *Never Let a Serious Crisis Go to Waste: How Neoliberalism Survived the Financial Meltdown*. London: Verso.

Mirowski, P. (2019) 'Hell Is Truth Seen Too Late' *boundary 2*, 46 (1): 1–53. https://doi.org/10.1215/01903659-7271327.

O'Shea, L. (2019) *Future Histories*. London: Verso.

Pfeil, F. (1993) 'Home Fires Burning, Family Noir in *Blue Velvet* and *Terminator 2*'. In J. Copjec (ed.), *Shades of Noir: A Reader*. London; New York: Verso.

Rothman, J. (2019) 'How William Gibson Keeps His Science Fiction Real'. *The New Yorker*, Dec.

Schrader, P. (2018a) *Transcendental Style in Film: Ozu, Bresson, Dreyer*. Oakland: University of California Press.

Schrader, P. (2018b) Transcript of lecture. https://www.bafta.org/media-centre/transcripts/bafta-screenwriters-lecture-series-paul-schrader.

Sterling, B. (2009) Gothic Chic in the Future Favela. http://mastersofmedia.hum.uva.nl/blog/2009/12/21/bruce-sterling-gothic-chic-in-the-future-favela/.

Taylor, A. (2019) *Democracy May Not Exist, But We'll Miss It When It's Gone*. London: Verso.

Thunberg, G. (2019) 'World Economic Forum'. *Davos*, 24 January.

Wasson, S. (2020) *The Big Goodbye: Chinatown and the Last Years of Hollywood*. Flatiron Books.

Wolfe, T. (1930) *God's Lonely Man*. Short novel, out of print.

6

SICARIO (VILLENEUVE, 2015)

The Rule of Law and the Terrorist State

Internal Worlds

At the beginning of the film the following is displayed, white on black:

> *The word Sicario comes from the zealots of Jerusalem.*
> *Killers who hunted the Romans who invaded their homeland.*
> *In Mexico, Sicario means hitman.*

There are zealots on both sides of the Mexican border whose dispute is over the control of and profit from the drug trade, economics rather than any religious concerns, even if the countries involved might self-identify as Catholic (Mexico) or Protestant (US).

The Mexican–American border as the repression barrier

If we treat the US as the conscious part of the self and Mexico as the unconscious part of the self and the border as the repression barrier, then Kate and Reggie are Federal Bureau of Investigation (FBI) operatives fighting to keep the USA 'sane' and governed by the rule of law against psychotic incursions from below the border. They are currently engaged in prosecuting such a fight against the Sonora drug cartel, who are apparently holding hostages in a house on a desert-fringed estate of tract housing in the outskirts of Phoenix. When they attack and enter the house, they find that all of the maimed and tortured hostages are dead, immured within the cavity walls. Whilst they are searching the house, a booby-trapped outhouse bomb is triggered, killing two of Kate's men. Kate and Reggie suffer minor injuries from the blast.

DOI: 10.4324/9781003206224-7

Literally and metaphorically sickened by this and conscious that she isn't making as much of a difference as she had hoped, Kate allows herself to be recruited for a new task force run by Matt, who we later discover is a Central Intelligence Agency (CIA) man. He, in turn, has employed Alejandro, the 'Sicario' or hitman, his 'bird-dog', whom we find out, works for a Colombian cartel. Their plan is to stir up trouble on the border and get the US representative of the Sonora cartel, Manuel Diaz, to go back to Mexico to meet with the third in charge of the cartel, Fausto, whose identity and location are currently unknown to Matt and Alejandro. This process has parallels with the therapeutic process for treating a hysterical symptom by tracing it back to the unconscious and expunging it by bringing it to consciousness.

After much cross-border subterfuge and provocation, Alejandro crosses the border into Mexico illegally and finds Fausto, killing both him and his family. All this in the hopes of moving the situation on the border back closer to the time of the Medellin – a powerful Colombian cartel which helped to keep the human and drug traffic across the border orderly by ensuring cooperation between Colombia, Mexico and the US, via agencies like the CIA. This move would in effect increase the efficiency of the repression barrier under the control of the CIA and the most powerful cartel. Alejandro, who was 'a man of the law' is coincidentally highly motivated by his need for revenge, as the Sonora cartel brutally and publicly killed his wife and daughter.

Endopsychic structure and the internal saboteur

The *Central* and *Ideal Selves* having been unable to stem the dreadful external, antilibidinal incursions from below the border, i.e., the unconscious, are open to receiving help from other internal self-systems like the preconscious *Libidinal* and *Antilibidinal Selves.*

In Fairbairn's original diagram (Figure 2.1) the unconscious antilibidinal ego is called the *Internal Saboteur.* Given the way that Matt and Alejandro treat Kate and Reggie throughout, one could argue that 'internal saboteur' is a more appropriate label than antilibidinal ego in this instance, since all of Matt and Alejandro's efforts are centred on sabotaging Kate and Reggie's synergy and effectiveness and achieving their own ends, that is, the ends of the CIA and the Colombian cartel who are the true unconscious *Antilibidinal Objects.*

Matt and Alejandro as internal *Antilibidinal Selves* that reject Reggie, an *Ideal Self* – because of his affiliation to the rule of law – get Kate, the *Central Self,* to voluntarily commit to their (undefined) cause on the promise of stemming the tide of external antilibidinal forces and making the repression barrier between the states stronger by punishing or removing the real perpetrators of the massacre that she and Reggie witnessed. That is, reducing the ability of the disruptive libidinal and antilibidinal forces to cross the repression barrier.

What they don't tell Kate is that they are going to operate without any regard for the rule of law; that they are going to agitate to engineer a further breakdown of this fragile barrier so they can get into Mexico and kill the leader of an external antilibidinal group, the Sonora cartel, in the interests of establishing control for a powerful Colombian antilibidinal group like the Medellin cartel, or their modern equivalent, in concert with the CIA so that they can take effective control of the border traffic.

They need Kate in order to legitimise the CIA activity on American soil and that is all. She is to be used to help cede control to the CIA and the stronger cartels and 'antilibidinal' international groups. When she threatens to tell everyone what actually went on, Alejandro threatens to kill her and make it look like suicide. She is forced, at gunpoint, to sign a paper stating they did everything 'by the book'. Alejandro treats her like a little girl, telling her disparagingly to go and find a small town where the rule of law still matters, since she will never survive on the border, which is now populated by wolves. She is angry enough to consider killing him and aims her service pistol at him as he walks away but cannot pull the trigger. She is broken.

Reggie has been broken earlier when someone he trusted, unbeknownst to him recruited by the Sonora cartel, tries to kill Kate. Alejandro, who had been following Kate since he is using her to 'bait the trap', comes to her rescue and saves her. She owes him her life. From this moment on, both the *Ideal* and the *Central Selves* are compromised, damaged, weakened and the *Antilibidinal Selves* are in the ascendency. Alejandro has extracted details from the cop of the location of the crossing and the names of anyone else in the police who is working for the cartel.

Libidinal Self

At first glance, there seems little room for the *Libidinal Self* as an explanatory concept in this analysis. It is true that Kate, driven by her *Libidinal Self*, gets involved with someone who could have killed her but whom she trusted because he was a friend of Reggie. This proved to be a significant part of her undoing and contributed to the loosening of the ties between Kate and Reggie, which was potentially their most important line of defence against Matt and Alejandro.

In Fairbairn's theory, the *Libidinal Self* is perennially under attack from the *Antilibidinal Self*, but it is not easy to see how this fits with the film until you remember Matt's diatribe against all of the people who are strongly motivated to buy the marijuana, cocaine and heroin and thus provide the impetus for the highly lucrative trade across the border. There is a strongly libidinal aspect of people's make-up that overrides their willingness to obey the rules of society. Matt acknowledges there is a huge demand, which he wants to be able to control for the mutual benefit of the CIA and the Colombian cartel, that is, to give them the power to control the supply and garner the profits that accrue from its sale. Reflecting his strongly antilibidinal sense of self, he is manifestly angry with people and their needs and denigrates them for their inability to control their need for the drugs. But the whole reason why the drugs are desirable, is libidinal; they bring pleasure. This may be a shallow pleasure, or even a self-destructive pleasure, but the strength of its appeal is the escapist pleasure it brings. These antilibidinal forces of 'law and order', which are ranged against the drug smugglers, are another manifestation of antilibidinal forces seeking to contain the libidinal forces of the pleasure seekers. In fact, the whole process of regulating the border is in essence an *Antilibidinal* attack upon the *Libidinal* writ large. The repressive antilibidinal aspect of government.

A solution for the 'War on Drugs' may well be to decriminalize the use of drugs – to allow the widespread legalisation of drugs for purchase and use, bringing them into the normal commercial environment from which governments could take their cut via taxes. It would also signal a change in mores towards a more openly 'libidinised' culture, which recent relaxation of the laws controlling the purchase and use of marijuana in the US would suggest is possible.

Intergenerational transmission and the repetition compulsion

There is a subtext running throughout the film concerning an ordinary Mexican state policeman who lives in relative poverty with his wife and their son. His son is mad on football and keeps worrying his father to play football with him.

This policeman, who is dirt poor, is also engaged in helping the cartel to smuggle drugs across the border to supplement his wages, using his patrol car for the purpose. When Alejandro identifies the tunnel, the cartels are using to smuggle drugs across the border, he hijacks this policeman and his car and then makes use of them to stop Manual Diaz on his way to see Fausto. When the policeman is no longer useful, Alejandro first kills him, and then kills Diaz as he gains access to Fausto's heavily guarded home in Mexico in order to execute him and his family.

At one point in this subplot, we see the boy going to touch his father's rifle and the policemen admonishing him. This poor boy, now without a father to guide him, impoverished and resentful, is likely to prove willing fodder if the cartel come recruiting in the future, thus continuing the never-ending cycle of violence.

For Fairbairn, the key to the repetition compulsion is internalised bad objects, and the brutal and unnecessary murder of this boy's father, like the brutal murder of Alejandro's wife and children and Alejandro's killing of Fausto and his family, will continue to feed the endless round of violence and destruction through generations to come.

In-group / Out-group

There are both in-groups and out-groups within the film and these change as the action of the film develops. Initially, Kate and Reggie are part of the same in-group – the FBI – posed against the out-group – the dominant Mexican cartels. Following their raid in Phoenix another in-group of nebulous origins – federal, national, international, DEA, CIA, it is never clear at this point – is formed and recruits Kate but excludes Reggie, probably because he is black and a trained lawyer. Once her acceptance has been reluctantly agreed to, Kate becomes an in-group member of a group that includes Kate, Matt and Alejandro. This in-group of Kate, Matt and Alejandro represent different structures within the political spectrum – FBI, CIA and a Colombian cartel – and are different endopsychic structures too – Kate is *Central Self* and Matt and Alejandro are *Antilibidinal Self* and object respectively. They are divided by their different attitudes towards the rule of law in general and in particular during this 'state of war', which is how Matt and Alejandro see it.

By marginalising Reggie, Matt makes Kate more dependent on himself and Alejandro. Both Kate and Reggie do their best to preserve their relationship and show a common front, but this is constantly undermined by both Matt and Alejandro. A determinate break is engineered by Alejandro, saving Kate from an attack by one of Reggie's 'friends', which makes her beholden to Alejandro. The main conflict within the central characters is based upon the fact there is a subgroup sympathetic to the CIA and Medellin cartel, and the law of the Talion (Matt, Alejandro), and a subgroup committed to the rule of law and mature dependence (Kate, Reggie). The law of the Talion, dog-eat-dog, subgroup, encourages chaos, provocation and retaliation, in order to convince the rule-of-law, mature-dependence subgroup, of the impossibility of a rational equitable and sensible political outcome under the rule of law. Hence, the deliberately inflammatory lightning raid across the border to bring a potential source across the border for interrogation on American soil, which is Kate's first independent, anxiety provoking, experience of the border.

The out-group is the Sonora cartel and all its operatives – Mexico in general and Juárez in particular. The assumption is that the out-group is nothing but torturing, murdering, assassins and drug smugglers. They are faceless, nightmarish creatures, never shown as normal, everyday people. The leaders of the Sonora cartel, Marco and Fausto are rich, respectable and unknown personally to Kate or Reggie; the other brother, Guillaume, is a prisoner and a convicted criminal who Matt and Alejandro spirit out of Juárez in order to get information on the crossing point they are going to raid and use. The ordinary policeman living in an impoverished border village is unknown to any of them, faceless, disposable, collateral damage, like the mutilated corpses that decorate cartel-controlled areas of Juárez, which seem like echoes from Goya's series of prints entitled *The Disasters of War*.

Overall Story

This is the story of how a person with a strong belief in the rule of law, who is a conscientious worker, and a conscious seeker after truth, and who is under extreme duress, can become damaged and broken by the machinations of internal *Antilibidinal* forces that sully the *Ideal Self* and brow beat, denigrate, lie to and deceive the *Central Self* whom they are only using to legitimate their illegal and unlawful activities. The main driver of this whole enterprise being revealed as revenge, power and profit, over and against the revenge, power and profit of another side, who are a mirror image, almost indistinguishable. The so-called law of the Talion, an eye for an eye, quite literally. The *Antilibidinal* control of the *Libidinal* for the benefit of the *Antilibidinal* forces, classical repression by a punitive super-ego using Freudian terms. A concerted attack on thinking it through, taking measured action, seeking to discuss and reach agreement, forcing the issue at the point of a gun, quite deliberately destructive of affording the space and time for thought and reason. Both sides of the border are composed of groups of battle hardened, heavily armed, men, waging war on each other in often brutal and callous ways without any higher-level intention or aim, which reflects the manifest failure at the political level to create a framework in which the smuggling of people and drugs is no longer a lucrative business.

To return to the analogy of the border being a repression barrier then; the attempts to control the flow of drugs and people across the border is like the efforts of the *Central* and *Ideal Selves* to prevent the transgressive *Libidinal* and *Antilibidinal Selves* from determining the body politic. It would be in the wider interests of all the states involved to strengthen the Mexican and Colombian states and make sure their economies were successful and not dependent upon drugs. All of which is anathema to capital and globalisation where the weak go to the wall and nationalism is the last refuge of a scoundrel.

In personal terms, it is about the rejection of attempts to move the border situation onto a rational basis under the rule of law and to maintain the chaos and the carnage that a state of war implies. It is about failing to move towards a mature approach to the problem and staying stuck in an infantile paranoid schizoid state. The triumph of vengeance, the Talion – an 'eye for an eye'; over reason – mature dependence, the proper recognition of difference.

External Worlds

The borders of Sicario

> Build a wall! Build a wall!

Trump's infamous rallying cry, partially built to little effect by the time of his defeat in 2020, is felt by its absence in Sicario. The wall here is porous. The enemy at the gate sits on both sides of the border.

Sicario is a film told through curtains and windows, in shades of blue and beige, set on an infamous geographical border (Mexico and the US), about the paper-thin line between law and lawlessness. It opens with an explosive crime and like Arthur Miller's great morality play *The Crucible*, it ends with a signature on a document to restore a so-called order – the state, capitalism, America, patriarchy – call it what you will. *Sicario* and the journey of its powerless protagonist, model FBI agent Kate Macer (Emily Blunt), reveal this order to be completely corrupt. The lie, and her enforced complicity, are necessary to maintain the veneer of truth around the activities of the American state and the CIA / Drugs Enforcement Agency. Throughout the film, lawlessness operates at a state level, and criminality is just a question of *Pirates and Emperors* (Noam Chomsky, 1986). The pirates in this case are the Mexican cartel; the emperors, the US government, as represented by their morally ambiguous black-ops department.

I saw *Sicario* in the *Grand Lumiere* at its World Premiere during the 2015 Cannes Film Festival. It feels important to remind myself of that. Looking back, it was a very different time, but the signs were already there to see, on screen at least. To paraphrase Gramsci, signs that the old world was crumbling and the new had not begun. Perhaps I was blind, and for the majority that world – "the beach beneath the pavement", the enlightenment, objective truth – had already gone, or worse still never really existed. But I still believe *Sicario* was one of those outlier films, the proverbial canary in the coal mine of the world to come for the West. Not just the West of Old America – New Mexico, California, Nevada and Arizona but the West of the Enlightenment – democracy, order and the idea that parents, on both sides of the border, would see better lives for their children. It prefigures the images of incarcerated children on the border that haunted the Trump administration mid-term and led Melania herself to momentarily break ranks with her husband's zero tolerance immigration policy.

Sicario clearly operates in a world where a moral compass might just kill you. It's interesting and significant that Rome is invoked in the title (and opening title legend). Life inside *Sicario*'s universe is neither black nor white, and the film eventually signals a creeping and largely hidden return to barbarism within the walls of Rome itself. Perhaps the film's greatest lesson is that life is cheap on either side of this border – regardless of who you are or were (and in fact it is this theme that is taken even further in its excellent sequel *Sicario 2: Day of the Soladado* (2018)). As Alejandro (Benicio del Toro), the Colombian lawyer cum assassin, the Sicario of the title, tells the persistent ingenue FBI agent Kate, that nothing will make sense to her American ears, and she will doubt everything that they do – but in the end she will understand. Understanding that the system is always the survivor and that people are merely collateral damage is the revelation in *Sicario*.

Sent on an unclear mission across the border to Juárez, Kate questions what they are actually doing. Frustrated she pleads for any information they can give her. But Alejandro fobs her off with a homily about a watch and how difficult it is to explain how it works, and recommends she just keep her eye on the time.

By the end of the film, she (and the audience) understands both the system (the watch) and the morality at play. Mentored by two bad father' – the shape-shifting of Alejandro and the criminality of Josh Brolin's ex-CIA Matt, she cannot entirely resist them. *Sicario* lives in a post-truth world where no one is bigger than the system and ultimately justice is just a liberal concept whose time has almost certainly passed.

Sicario's universe is a prescient warning of the world to come post-Trump. A post-truth world unveiled and unmasked further during the pandemic. The pandemic being a particular moment of unveiling, where we have learnt that domestic American life is as expendable and cheap as any other – whether in the service of protecting the wealth and economy of the US (via Border Control and the War on Drugs) or by building an imaginary / imagined Trumpian wall, or in service to some spurious question of 'herd immunity' or 'business as usual'.

Writing this in 2020, even without the current pandemic, five years seems like a lifetime ago in both film and politics. Obama was still in the White House; Trump had not even declared himself a serious candidate or invoked the idea of "building a wall" and the 'War on Terror' in the Middle East felt like it was drifting to an uneasy close as America withdrew troops from Iraq and Afghanistan – another failed foreign excursion in US foreign policy and the 'War on Terror'.

History will remember these Middle East Crusades best perhaps as a successful invocation of the law of the Talion (revenge for 9/11) but also as a complete disaster for the region and ultimately America. The twenty-first century saw a flurry of conflict-based Hollywood films from *Rendition* and *Hurt Locker* to *Green Zone* and *Zero Dark Thirty.* Like their Vietnamese War–based predecessors, these were all told from an exclusively American point of view – there is only 'the other' in this cinema of incursion. Like Trump himself, *Sicario* turned inwards to look at the enemy at the gate – most popularly embodied and named here and in shows like *Narcos* or *Queen of the South* as 'the cartel'.

Villeneuve the Auteur

It is worth noting that Denis Villeneuve's film before this was *Prisoners* – a film that glances back at the ghosts of American torture abroad, relocated to a domestic and religious setting. For Villeneuve, in *Prisoners*, the post-9/11 world of war is coming home to roost. Mass slaughter, war and drone strikes abroad – these were policies instigated by a Republican President Bush and re-enforced with a different but still brutal policy by President Obama. Trump took a very different, insular, view of American foreign policy. For him, America needed to focus its power and military might on its immediate surroundings.

Twenty-fifteen was also a different place for film-makers where a mini-studio could still make an intelligent genre film (a $30 million budget) and also turn a profit. Netflix was only available in the Americas and Europe (it expanded to its current 192 countries through 2016) and stood at less than half its current subscription base, and larger indies like *Lionsgate* were still thriving. It was indeed normal and fiscally sound to make *Sicario* for theatrical release and without the backing of a streamer.

For Villeneuve, off the back of the critically lauded *Incendies* and the commercially successful *Prisoners* (and brilliant 'doubles' movie *Enemy),* *Sicario* signalled his arrival at that rare table – the thinking man's commercial / genre auteur who could became a 'brand'. With the success of *Sicario*, Villeneuve hit his stride, and from *Prisoners* through to the *Dune* adaptation, made five big movies in seven years, working with the biggest stars of the day – from Ryan Gosling, Emily Blunt and Timothée Chalamet, to Jake Gyllenhaal, Amy Adams and Josh Brolin.

Undoubtedly now, Chris Nolan and Villeneuve stand alone, as the Spielberg and Ridley Scott of this decade – few are trusted with such projects so regularly or given the option to pick and choose with huge budgets. After *Sicario*, Villeneuve's next three films clocked in at budgets of $50–$200 million, as studios allowed him to bet much bigger. Thematically, he took a journey of scale and time from the tiny, short taxi driver / director story in 1998's *Cosmos* through the current political moment – *Incendies* in the Middle East / Canada, *Prisoners* in America, *Sicario* on the Mexican border – all deal with the wars on terror and drugs in their own way – all thrillers in their own style, to stories that reach beyond this Earth into unknown futures and alien worlds.

Sicario opens with a rolling, driving bass line. Villeneuve used *Jaws* as temp music whilst editing the film. His composer, the now deceased Johan Johannsson, then brilliantly almost 'out-Jawsed' that seminal John Williams soundtrack throughout the film's set pieces. The film opens with Johannsson's bone-cracking bass line, followed by the aforementioned title text explaining the Roman origin of the word Sicario, self-aggrandising and mythologising this story and simultaneously invoking the explanatory cards at the beginning of Ridley Scott's *Blade Runner* (1982). This is followed by an opening shot of a very beige American suburbia. An image from Spielberg's *ET*, but washed out. The suburb is disturbed by military personnel in black, and we then cut to the face of Kate (Emily Blunt) and Ronnie (Daniel Kaluuya). They are both sat in an armoured truck in full ultra-militarised uniform and gear.

They crash through the wall of a suburban house in an armoured vehicle and a flurry of machine gun fire. This is no ordinary suburban home – embedded in the walls of this house, like the Capuchin Crypt in Rome – lie the dead themselves, victims of the cartel. The bodies of their victims are literally buried in and behind the walls. Villeneuve uses lingering (Francis) Baconesque close-ups of disfigured faces like the macabre emaciated 'Sloth' victim from Fincher's *Seven*. When asked what to tell her superiors, Kate merely replies, "the truth". Like Polanski's *Chinatown* sleuth Jake Gittes, looking for the truth and caring about it is exactly what will get Kate into trouble. This Arizona sequence ends with part of the house exploding in a booby trap set by the cartel, invoking Jonathan Demme's *Silence of the Lambs* and the decoy booby trapped house that explodes toward the end of that film.

In the space of a little over five minutes, via this FBI raid on a drugs house, Villeneuve invokes half a dozen of the greatest genre films of the last 35 years. Suburbia is no longer the safe home of the broken but warm families of *ET* and Jake Gittes and Clarissa Starling are transmuted into the body of another young FBI agent Kate. This is all underscored by an ever-ominous *Jaws* like soundtrack and chilling imagery like *Seven*. It is the Arizona of 2015, but like William Gibson's aphorism – this is both future and present – and as unevenly distributed as it could possibly be. We are in the borderlands between horror and sci-fi, between stylised action and political thriller, between truth and fiction, between the behemoth US and its weaker neighbour Mexico.

We are in a world we no longer recognise, the horror of suburbia as invoked in Lynch's lush *Blue Velvet* picket fence world is replaced by the cartel's innocuous sand-coloured house. Secrets don't lie in severed ears in the grass here, but beneath plasterboard and dusty basements. Even in the relative Americana familiarity of Arizona, we are immediately in another country. A hinterland where the rule of law is under extreme scrutiny and the law of the Talion is the driver for at least one of our protagonists.

The Edge of Truth

Sicario's modern morality play is foregrounded with the featuring throughout of the American flag alongside Kate. As the ethical lines become blurred, the flag becomes less seen. The presence of the flag as a symbol (of power), is much the same way as we see it used in *First Reformed*, always placed significantly in frame. The palette of *Sicario* is outlined in the excellent video essay, *Sicario – The Mirage of a Moral World* (Digging Deeper, 2016).

> Villeneuve and Deakins chose different colors to represent certain ideals of morality, like blue for justice, black for corruption, and beige for the true morally ambiguous nature of human beings without labels. We see the storytelling power of color in the protagonist Kate. In the beginning of the film, she wears bold blue colors, but as time goes on, it gets desaturated to a bluish grey.

Veteran cinematographer Roger Deakins and Villeneuve work on wide lenses at high-tension moments – moments normal Hollywood films would go to medium shots and close-ups. Their use of windows and wide shots gives us both a sense of watching something that we can't quite see and watching something that is real – a realist documentary style almost. Like most aspects of the film, it's very deliberate and precise, and the message of an amoral lawless real world is very clear. We are always on the edge of truth, embedded in fiction.

Sicario goes on to tell Agent Kate's story, as she is recruited into an 'inter agency task force' to work with the CIA by Brolin's shady character Matt Graver, and Alejandro, a former lawyer turned assassin (the Sicario of the title). Their aim is to cut the head off of the cartel and take down the "men who are really responsible for today", today being the explosion in the booby-trapped house which kills some of Kate's FBI compatriots. Mid-way through the film, as she discovers the real mission and who these men are, Alejandro tells her "Every Day … he [the head of the cartel] kills…. To find him would be like finding a vaccine". But eventually Kate discovers she has been recruited essentially as a 'beard' for a series of black-ops border incursions that are told in the two major set pieces of the film. She is the patsy that allows Graver, the CIA head of the operation, to do what he does. And what he does is clearly a form of state terrorism.

When we meet Graver, he is in beige, the only non-suited man at a table of Kate's formally dressed superiors. She is initially separated from him by thick sound-proof glass, one of many such borders that are both translucent but impenetrable. He is marked out by his casual surfer-style long hair and sandals (the close-up shot of his bare feet is given time here by Villeneuve's lingering camera). He could clearly pass for a Silicon Valley disruptor or a *Vice* magazine editor – but we realise very quickly he is neither. Following on from Jameson's 1977 seminal essay 'Class and Allegory in Contemporary Culture: Dog Day Afternoon as Political Film', Graver can be seen as one of the new representatives of capitalism. Whilst globalised capital is hard to physically locate and identify and Jameson saw this even in 1977, the new Silicon Valley Burning Man class of 2015 – the new billionaire class – the Bezos's, the Musks, the Zuckerbergs are clearly recognisable in Graver's uniform of neutral colours, open-toed sandals, long hair and casual attire. This attire was originally the signifier of a counter-cultural figure from the late 1960s. The Haight-Ashbury circle of San Francisco gentrification completes itself as the stoner Dude with an AK-47 – the signifier can no longer be trusted in the chain of signification. Graver, like Elon Musk or Travis Kalacnik, becomes the post-modern wolf in sheep's clothing, a signifier who has swopped its hippy leanings for some darker purpose.

This shifting around subcultures, the ability for mainstream culture to absorb that which it at first is antagonistic to, is one of the features of postmodernism that explains Trump and other populist movements. As Matthew Flisfeder puts it:

> In the postmodernist society of the spectacle appearance matters more than essence and, in this primacy, given to the superficial, those ideas to which modernism found itself devoted, such as depth, originality and novelty seem to perish. The punk rock politics of "anarchy in the UK" descends into a mere fashion decision.
>
> *(Flisfeder, 2017, p. 153)*

Examining the impact of this on modern politics he observes:

> if all resistance can now be accommodated by the mainstream – if resistance in other words is now part of the mainstream … what remains of the ability to resist the official culture? … something peculiar begins to occur: the conservative Right starts to look increasingly like the only radical alternative to dominant culture – hence we also see the rise of the new Right and neo-conservatism arriving in parallel with the emergence of postmodernism … itself using images and themes of rebellion to appeal to the masses, making it appear as the Right is a truly counter-hegemonic force … The politics of postmodernism, I claim, are therefore a decontextualized "politics without politics". Without the necessary historical context and background of postmodern theory its politics risk dissolving into commercialism, right wing populism or cynical resignation.
>
> *(ibid., p. 27)*

For much of the period 2015–2020 we saw evidence of all three. As we see with Graver initially – surfaces matter more than depth. But the film goes on to examine what lies beneath the veneer of blue and beige, the proto-hippy casual style. After the intro of Graver, Kate is taken to a black-ops meeting near the border. Here we see Graver change even more as he briefs the mission. The exchanges between him and the motley crew of agents, military and mercenary militia (a 'coalition of the willing' to coin George Bush's phrase) takes in quips about sexually transmitted diseases, terrorists in Fiji, ex-Afghanistan veterans, prison jokes and Matt's drinking problem. Kate is clearly not part of the Boys' Club on show here. Later in the film, this male-dominated patriarchal world becomes more threatening than mere lewd barroom advice. The first person that tries to kill Kate is a cartel member in the Arizona death house during the opening, the second a gang member on the border during her first 'mission' for Graver. But more frighteningly still, the third attempt is by a man she invites into her own home. In a 'honey trap', in a bar back in Phoenix (after she rashly and naïvely identifies herself by going into a bank and getting ID'ed on CCTV) she is rescued from a murder attempt in her own home by Alejandro, who has been tracking her.

Later, on two separate occasions, a gun is pointed at her by Alejandro himself – first in Mexico and then at the denouement in her own home again. If it isn't clear from the first frame that Kate's life is in danger whatever side of the border she's on or whatever side she takes, by the last, it patently is. Even domestic life is no guarantee of safety anymore.

Essentially, Matt Graver entices Kate into the male-dominated world of beige to cover his operation with the feminine blue-black veneer of her FBI / DEA authority. He needs to disguise himself and his black-ops, to hide as the wolves in plain sight. The maleness and racism of this world (Kate's sympathetic partner Reggie, and her only friend, it seems, is African American) is seen most pointedly when, just before the first foray into Mexico, we see Alejandro take off his beige jacket and place it carefully in a blue bag. This quiet moment of preparation is a clear metaphor for the two uniforms these wolves wear – the beige casual jacket that allows them to operate without moral compass and the blue cover of the rule of law. This blue veil is their alibi, their enabler, and Kate is its representative.

In *Sicario*'s War on Drugs narrative, a Mexican civil policeman and his son in Juárez are given some small beats throughout the film. They feel disconnected from the main story, but they show us life on the other side of the border. The cop – a good guy with his child, a decent man in blue turns out to be a cog in the wheel of the cartel 'watch'. When Alejandro faces him, he has no hesitation in killing him, like any other criminal. Nothing must get in the way of Alejandro's revenge, including the law.

The final shot of the movie then returns to Juárez and the policeman's little boy – he is playing football on a dirt pitch by a high-security fence – a whistle starts the game, the pitch is marked out, the teams are in clear colours – green and yellow – colours we have rarely seen in this film. This is a game with rules, but their simple game is punctuated by automatic gunfire in the near distance. It is clear that, for these children, the adult world, the drug world, a dangerous game without rules continues close by.

Conclusion

Early on in Sicario when asked what she wants from a colleague, as she stands in her blue DEA uniform, Kate answers, "the truth". And it is this search for the truth that leads her across the border (twice) and into the lawlessness of Mexico. But the real message of *Sicario* is that the law on both sides of the border is broken and that the War on Drugs is as corrupt and vengeful as the cartel.

By the end of the film, Kate has discovered that the 'watch' Alejandro referenced earlier is built on lies. He tells her, having clearly threatened her life to ensure the safety of this mission and future ones, that she should retire to a small town where the rule of law still exists, since she will never survive on the frontier since she is not a wolf, and the frontier is the land of wolves.

We come to realise there is no vaccine for these ills – only revenge. The 'watch' Alejandro references when he first talks to her is complex but tells only a subjective reality / time – an amoral American ideology rather than an objective reality. We and eventually Kate understand that the law is dead, and Kate is merely an expendable pawn in this lawless game.

Perhaps what *Sicario* really unveils, though, is that what is revealed in the Trump years is a more extreme and transparent continuation of what we already knew even during the Obama years – that American aggression goes largely unchecked throughout the world, the CIA operates with impunity and the American economy is primary. Human life, American or not, is just the collateral damage of the nation's drive for wealth and power.

What *Sicario* foretells is that America's new war is not only on its borders but is an old war re-pitched – a war with itself. The power of a woman within the American Dream is insignificant, minute. The 'watch' has stopped. The law is meaningless. And the time is always the same. An unending, unlawful struggle to keep the drugs flowing, the money protected and America supreme.

References

Chomsky, N. (1986) *Pirates and Emperors, Old and New Version*, New Edition. London: Pluto Press.

Digging Deeper (2016) 'Sicario: The Mirage of a Moral World'. https://www.youtube.com/watch?v=0nrjHF7wPbs (last accessed 25 June 2020).

Flisfeder, M. (2017) *Postmodern Theory and Blade Runner*. London: Bloomsbury.

Jameson, F. (1992) 'Class and Allegory in Contemporary Culture: *Dog Day Afternoon* as Political Film.' In *Signatures of the Visible*, 1st edition. New York: Routledge.

7

JOKER (PHILLIPS, 2019)

Put on a Happy Face

Internal Worlds

Origins

Joker is a 'just so' story, a story of origins. A 'How the leopard got its spots' sort of tale, but in this case "'a tale told by an idiot, full of sound and fury signifying nothing". The narrator is unreliable, and so is the narrative. This is a fractured account both of the day-to-day and the past, and very possibly the future too. Joker, before he becomes the Joker, is an impoverished, mentally ill man, Arthur Fleck, who was badly abused as a child, and is now living in poverty with his demented mother. He is a man who has been treated for mental illness previously and is still taking seven medications for his condition and seeing a counsellor. His 'condition' is not clear, but on the evidence is probably what is often called 'borderline personality'. What is described as his condition, the presenting symptom as it were, is a mirthless laugh at times of uncertainty, stress and anxiety. This is probably the consequence of childhood beatings and abuse when he was three, of which he is unaware, which run counter to his mother's assertions that he was a happy little boy. He is also unaware that he was adopted and that it was his mother's boyfriend who caused the abuse, while she sat idly by, for which she was hospitalised and lobotomised. He is totally confused about his father, since his mother insists that he is big businessman Thomas Wayne's bastard. This has been denied by Wayne, his family and advisors, despite the photo of Penny, Arthur's mother, with a note from a 'TW' on the back, saying how beautiful she looks. Unreliable narrators, unreliable narratives – if, as Winnicott says, therapy is a matter of history-taking, then there are numerous impediments to therapy here since the history-taking is occluded, fractured, partial and unreliable.

DOI: 10.4324/9781003206224-8

As for his originally adopting the identity of a clown, who eventually transmutes into *Joker*, this might have been prompted by Wayne's public comments about the ordinary people protesting on the street being clowns, or in a common American epithet for men or friends 'you jokers'. But, at the beginning of the film he is already depicted as dressing and performing as a clown to make a living, which perhaps has parallels with carnivalisation (Bakhtin, 1982) and 'carny' folk, as a suitable occupation for a liminal figure, an outsider, divorced even from himself. This could also be related to the trickster figure in mythology.

> Many native traditions held clowns and tricksters as essential to any contact with the sacred. People could not pray until they had laughed, because laughter opens and frees from rigid preconception. Humans had to have tricksters within the most sacred ceremonies for fear that they forget the sacred comes through upset, reversal, surprise. The trickster in most native traditions is essential to creation, to birth.
>
> *(Gibbens, 2001)*

The actual transformation from clown and possible stand-up comic into *Joker* follows from four connected experiences. (a) Arthur's murder of three Wall Street types on the 'El'; (b) his realising that his 'girlfriend' is a figment of his imagination; (c) his finding out about his mother, Penny, and the past he has suffered; and (d) lastly, his killing of his mother. "So farewell hope, and with hope farewell fear, Farewell remorse; all good to me is lost. Evil, be thou my good" (Milton, 1674). This is a transformation which Fairbairn discusses when talking about the *Moral Defence*:

> In a world ruled by the Devil the individual may escape the badness of being a sinner; but he is bad because the world around him is bad. Further, he can have no sense of security and no hope of redemption. The only prospect is one of death and destruction.
>
> *(Fairbairn, 1952, p. 67)*

Developmentally, Arthur was a three-year-old child, at about the time that his mother was sectioned, and he was beaten and abused by her boyfriend, which places him, and his experience of abuse, in the period after the basic endopsychic structure was becoming established, and it remains pre-oedipal, an unresolved and unstable part of the transitional period in Fairbairn's developmental schema. It also suggests that *Joker* sees himself as the devil or has taken on the idea that the world is actually ruled by the devil, of which he is an embodiment. (See later section on the The Devil and the Joker.)

> since the joy of loving seems hopelessly barred to him, he may as well deliver himself over to the joy of hating and obtain what satisfaction he

> can out of that. He thus makes a pact with the Devil and says, 'Evil be thou my good'. The moral motive is determined by the consideration that, if loving involves destroying, it is better to destroy by hate, which is overtly destructive and bad, than to destroy by love which is by rights creative and good.
>
> *(Fairbairn, 1952, p. 27)*

Story

We first see Arthur Fleck as he is putting on clown make-up in the dressing room of 'Ha-Ha', a company that hires clowns out to various businesses and gatherings. Throughout the opening of *Joker*, we follow Arthur as he tries to make a living as a clown in a Gotham City that looks like the US during the depression. Arthur suffers from some sort of hysterical condition that provokes mirthless laughter when he is embarrassed or anxious; he is an awkward misfit.

In the opening hour of *Joker*, we see the lead character, Arthur, working at a 'clown for hire' agency and taking random jobs. Gotham City is a world in meltdown, with widespread poverty and unemployment, uncollected rubbish on the streets, vermin and dereliction. While advertising a closing down sale, his advertising sign is stolen by a group of youths. When he takes chase and catches them, they turn on him and brutally beat him .

Arthur is not well liked by the 'Ha-Ha' company boss and is threatened with the sack for losing the advertising sign. One of his fellow 'clowns for hire', forces a gun and ammunition on him, 'for self-protection'. Arthur takes the gun with him to the children's ward of a hospital, where he is working as a clown to lift the spirits of the kids, but accidentally drops the gun on the floor, which frightens both the kids and the staff. He is sacked from his job at 'Ha-Ha' as a consequence.

On his way back home on the empty and dirty subway, he witnesses a group of 'city types' molesting a girl and, after accidentally provoking them by his laugh so that they attack, and beat and kick him, like the youths who stole the sign did, he shoots the three of them dead, and runs off home. In the lavatory of his tenement block, he dances narcissistically to his reflection in the mirror. Meanwhile and throughout the film, society is in meltdown, people are out of work, poverty-stricken and angry. There is widespread protest on the streets. After the murder of the three 'yuppies' on the subway by a clown, many of the protesters adopt clown masks or make-up.

Arthur's mother is ill and cared for by Arthur. Arthur, who is on 'welfare', is attempting to support them both, living together in a rundown tenement block, by working at the comedy venues. There is an attractive young black woman with a little girl who lives in the same block in an adjacent apartment who seems to strike up a relationship with Arthur when they meet in a lift.

Arthur's mother is obsessed with big businessman and local leading politician Thomas Wayne (the future Batman's father), who she worked with over 30 years ago before she became sick, and claims that he fathered her child, i.e., Arthur.

While watching a TV show hosted by Murray Franklin (Robert De Niro) with his mother, Arthur imagines himself as an audience member of the show. In his fantasy, he comes to the attention of the host because of his strange laugh, and is then 'recognised' by the host who thinks there is something special about him. When Murray talks about his own father deserting his family, Arthur says that he has been the man of the house for as long as he can remember, and that he has taken good care of his mother. He says that she always told him to smile, to put on a happy face, and that he was put here to spread joy and laughter. Arthur is brought on stage, and when they go to the commercial break Murray says he'd give up all the glitz and the glamour in a heartbeat to have a kid like him. They hug, and Arthur, who is desperate for a father, is deeply moved.

Arthur thinks he might have a career as a stand-up comedian and goes to a comedy store with the young woman neighbour to try out his material, which he carries around with him in a dog-eared notebook containing material like, "I hope my death makes more *cents* than my life." Most of his dealings with this young woman neighbour are portrayed realistically but turn out to be his fantasy.

Arthur's mother writes to Thomas Wayne, but Arthur reads the letter before it is sent. The letter is a grovelling embarrassment, pleading for Wayne to help her and 'their' kid. Incensed, Arthur goes to see Wayne at his mansion and accidentally meets a young Bruce Wayne (the future Batman). Arthur is told by the Waynes' butler that his mother, Penny, is delusional, was committed to an asylum and that Wayne has nothing to do with him or his mother, and to get lost.

Arthur goes to check what he has been told and steals his mother's medical records from the Arkham Asylum, discovering that he was adopted and that his mother was suffering from some mental illness and that, when he was three, she let one of her boyfriend's beat and abuse Arthur, whose present condition is probably due to that abuse. Arthur goes to the hospital where his mother has been taken, suffering from a suspected heart attack brought on by the police when they visited recently to ask about Arthur and the subway killings. Arthur suffocates his mother because she betrayed him and lied to him for years. He has come to the realisation that he hasn't been happy for even one minute of his entire life.

Murray Franklin, the TV host, plays a clip from Arthur's performance at the comedy store in order to poke fun, but is surprised when there is a popular call for him to have Arthur appear on the show. Arthur is invited to go on the show, and while he is getting prepared, applying the clown face, dying his hair green, etc., two of the people from 'Ha-Ha' come to commiserate with him, having heard that his mother has died. He brutally kills the one who had given him the gun in order to entrap him, but lets the other one go, a 'little person', who was always kind to him.

Now fully identified as Joker, he goes to join the protest in the streets on his way to the TV studio, to appear on Murray Franklin's show. He manages to escape the two cops who are on his tail, and in the melee on the streets and in the subway both the cops get beaten up by the, by now out of control, crowds, most of whom are dressed as clowns. As he is fleeing the cops down a long flight of steps in full *Joker* regalia, the soundtrack plays Gary Glitter's 'Rock and Roll Part 2' to accompany his narcissistic dancing.

When Arthur gets to the TV studio, he insists that he is introduced as 'Joker', at which point he dances in to the studio and passionately and inappropriately kisses an old woman psychiatrist before turning to be interviewed by Murray.

Murray at first tries to distance Arthur / Joker from the riots in the street, but Arthur incriminates himself by confessing to killing the Wall Street types before shooting Murray in cold blood and accusing him of just wanting to make fun of him.

Joker leaves the studio and joins the rioting clowns on the streets of Gotham. The soundtrack has Cream playing 'White Room' as the mayhem on the streets is revealed.

Meanwhile, Thomas Wayne and his wife are taking young Bruce back home from the theatre when a clown shoots them both dead, leaving Bruce Wayne (Batman) an orphan.

The cops catch Joker, but an ambulance, driven by a clown, crashes into the cop car and two 'clowns' rescue Joker and lay him out on the hood of the cop car like a fallen hero. As Joker revives and struggles to stand, he revels in the chaos he sees around him, and starts to dance as the crowd around him go wild. He is like a god dancing the destruction of the world around him. A Shiva, a Kali?

The next we see of him, Joker is back inside an asylum being interviewed by the same actor who played the social worker earlier on, but this time she is a much more upmarket psychiatrist. She asks him what is so funny as he laughs his laugh, and he says he was thinking of a joke, which is accompanied by a shot of young Bruce Wayne standing in an alley next to his dead parents. Joker says that she wouldn't get it and starts to sing 'That's Life', Murray's theme song. The last shots of the film show him running down a corridor of the asylum leaving a trail of bloody footprints, being pursued by unknown others.

Analysis

If we accept that the putative *Central Self* is Arthur, then we start with a very damaged self, an abused child with a condition, a clown doing badly paid work in an impoverished environment, with his damaged mother as his *Ideal Self* whom he looks after diligently, despite their poverty and her dementia.

He meets a *Libidinal Self* in the form of a young woman and her daughter living down the hall, who appears to warm to him which prompts, and encourages him, in fantasy at least, to become braver and more active.

He believes his mother's story that Thomas Wayne is his father, but a bad father who will not help his mother or support his son who needs him. Meanwhile TV talk show host Murray Franklin is an 'adopted' good father.

Because of the accidental revelation in the children's ward that he has a gun, which was given him by another bad father figure, Arthur loses his job. The antilibidinal activity of the Wall Street guys leads to his shooting them as a protector of another possible *Libidinal Self*, a young woman, which makes him feel better about himself. The *Central Self* has overcome some aspects of the *Antilibidinal Self*'s attack on the *Libidinal Self* and deserves to be rewarded by the *Libidinal Self*, which is why, after killing the Wall Street guys, Joker dances grandiosely in front of the mirror in a sort of narcissistic celebration inflating his *Ideal Self*. He then goes to see the young woman who lives down the hall, who it is implied willingly goes to bed with him, but which we see later is also just fantasy. His *Central Self* has been empowered, and he goes to the comedy store and performs, accompanied by the young woman (the *Central Self* and the *Libidinal Self* in alliance, which is again fantasy).

Finding a grovelling letter that his mother is about to send to Thomas Wayne, he decides to find out the truth and plead for Penny, his mother, to be looked after by Wayne. In the end, he finds out that Penny has been lying to him about his parentage and is herself partly responsible for his condition.

His *Ideal Self* is in tatters, so he goes to see his *Libidinal Object*, who it turns out is much more fantasy than real. He kills his mother as *Ideal Object* and is no longer able to sustain a relationship with the girl down the hall as *Libidinal Self*. This leaves his own impoverished *Central Self*, the one that killed the stockbrokers exposed and unstable. The polar opposite of the bad father, is Wayne, who branded Joker and everyone like him as clowns in an election speech he made on TV saying that people like himself who have made something of themselves will always look at those who haven't as nothing but clowns. The neoliberal 'entrepreneur of one's own soul' ideology writ large. Joker adopts the badge of clown with pride and makes it a badge of honour. He elevates his clown self to be his true self and regresses to an *Antilibidinal Self / Internal Saboteur*, 'Evil be my good' and becomes Joker.

Joker, as destroyer of all things, echoing Oppenheimer's words from the Bhagavad Gita. "Now I am become death, the destroyer of worlds." The lord of misrule. A practising nihilist, "I don't believe in anything", as he says on the TV show, before murdering Murray for exploiting him, changing Murray from a good to a bad father 'in a heartbeat'.

Driven mad by big business, political power structures and the dog-eat-dog world of neoliberal, individualist ideology, he wants to see the whole society explode in flames and destroy itself. He is an undeveloped self, an infantile self, unable to internalise anything positive from his environment, alone and vulnerable, on the border between the neurotic and the psychotic, close to total fragmentation and madness. Forever excluded from the American Dream, he can only revel in its apparent destruction.

The Devil and the Joker

The early environmental failure that left Arthur a deeply disturbed little boy and prevented him from maturing developmentally, left him at the stage of *Infantile Dependence* with only weakly established endopsychic structures. His attempts at growing up are forever frustrated by his need to look after his sick mother.

His attempts to use the *Moral Defence* have never been properly carried through, so that his mother is both a good mother and a bad mother and these two are intimately tied to two possible fathers – Murray Franklin as a good father, and Thomas Wayne as a bad father.

Mostly he is a good boy, who looks after his good mother in their impoverished lives while she, as a bad mother, obsesses about her rich ex-boss who she claims is Arthur's real father and should support them but won't because he is a bad father. Meanwhile Arthur and Penny enjoy the little pleasure that Murray Franklin as a good father brings through his TV show, which they watch together as Arthur looks after his good mother to the best of his abilities.

I want to introduce here the idea that the chaos into which Joker propels Gotham City is the equivalent to what Janine Chasseguet-Smirgel calls "the destruction of reality". It is not possible to explore this here in great depth, but it is interesting to note that Joker does revel in his killing of the young men whilst in the lavatory of his own tenement, and that he confronts Thomas Wayne in the lavatory of a 'swanky' hotel.

For Chasseguet-Smirgel (1991), reality "from a psychosexual perspective may be defined as resulting from the existence of the father separating the mother and child", something that has not been available to Joker. She goes on to suggest that "reality is recognition of sexual and generational differences", which have likewise been unavailable to Joker. "Or, yet again: mother and father have a procreative sexuality, whereas the child does not." And Joker, as a man, does not have this either. This leads on to the idea that the destruction of reality is equivalent to destruction of the paternal universe. Chasseguet-Smirgel discusses some clinical cases:

> one of which centers on the assassination of an old man who, besides representing a paternal oedipal image, also represents reality itself. This case illustrates in concrete form the murder of the father, and hence of reality, accomplished by the pervert when he eradicates the paternal dimension of psychosexuality by regressing to the anal sadomasochistic dimension.
>
> *(Chasseguet-Smirgel, 1991, p. 399)*

While there are few obvious signs of sadomasochism in the way the Joker is portrayed in the film, a deep understanding of what he has become through the negligence and abuse of his early upbringing, taken together with his execution of Murray Franklin, may suggest that he is indeed deeply regressed.

> The object is to act out a fantasy of revenge which transforms an infantile trauma into an adult triumph … I believe, in fact, that the perversions sweep the *genital dimensio*n of human sexuality from the scene, or, to put it another way, the very idea of fertile adult sexuality, i.e., the sexuality of the parents, is denied and abolished. The pervert's hatred is aimed at reality in general. This is essentially composed of differences … differences between man and woman, child and adult, between the appearance of the need (or the wish) and its satisfaction. In short, acceptance of reality, for the small boy… means acknowledging the need to wait until he has the psychosexual maturity to satisfy an adult woman (a substitute for the mother) and to give her a child. This means admitting the need to grow, to develop, and to identify with the father in order, like him, to possess a fertilizing genital penis. This is to admit that the father is endowed with prerogatives that the child will only acquire later; it is acceptance of the fact that the genital primal scene and the adult's powers of procreation lie beyond the child's reach.
>
> *(Chasseguet-Smirgel, 1991, p. 401)*

In a different but related paper, Chasseguet-Smirgel (1999) draws attention to Freud's view that "The basic idea is that perversions are equivalent to 'Devil Religions'". She continues:

> In viewing perversion as a 'Devil religion', we find two concepts of the devil, the one relating to anality and the other to the 'Luciferian' idea of the devil, the 'bearer of light' who snatched a spark of God's fire, the fallen angel who rebelled against the Creator.
>
> *(Chasseguet-Smirgel, 1999, p. 383)*

I am struck here by the mention of a 'spark of fire', which is of course the main way in which the revolt by the 'clowns' is represented in the film as a citywide conflagration. Later in the same paper, she goes on to delineate a common "background of anal-sadistic regression" whose aim "is to destroy reality, composed of differences and in its place to establish the reign of anality where all the differences have been abolished" (ibid., p. 385) Quite the opposite of *Mature Dependence*, in which differences that make a difference (Bateson) are crucial. Joker is in fact the exemplary superhero, deeply flawed, a grandiose, narcissistic Nietzschean, Übermensch, who generates his own inhuman, amoral, values, rather than complying with other's values, and who destroys the ability to differentiate, reducing everything to an undifferentiated anal bolus. From a Fairbairnian perspective he is, like Trump, a personification of the *Internal Saboteur*, or more strikingly represents the inability to emerge from an infantile dependency that destroys reality and reduces everything to shit.

External Worlds

An age of heroes

> Is it me or is it just getting crazier out there?
>
> *(Arthur Fleck aka Joker)*

To say that we are living in the age of superhero films is no exaggeration. Strong arguments have been made about the comfortable fit between the transnational nature of narrative world building and neoliberalism. In 2021, we are completely *au fait* with imaginary worlds that operate not only "in media but across it". When built right, multiplatform universes – Star Wars, Marvel, DC, Game of Thrones, Harry Potter et al. – are the "sure thing" for the risk-averse behemoth studios. Of all the companies that has understood this best, Disney stands out from the crowd, having made two huge purchases of intellectual property – Marvel Comics in 2009 and Star Wars in 2012 for $4 billion each. In the last decade they have gone on to generate more than $15 billion in income for Disney and are now integral to its assault on the streaming world, with Disney+ looking set to overtake Netflix's subscription numbers and become the biggest streamer by 2024.

We could devote a book to the many crossing points between neoliberalism and the superhero genre – both in form, production and dissemination. In his earlier work *Capitalist Superheroes* (2012), Dan Hassler-Forest took the stance that,

> the superhero movie genre … has maintained its central position within contemporary popular culture … Even as critical voices continue to predict that the now ten-year-old phenomenon of the superhero movie must finally be nearing its end.

Nearly a decade later, superhero movies and TV shows continue to grow. In fact, during Trump's presidency, the genre became bigger and more dominant in terms of its box office and market domination. As Spencer (2018) says, "In 2017, seven of the 20 highest-grossing domestic films were superhero movies." It wasn't a huge leap to see how, back in 2018,

> the tenets of neoliberalism fit perfectly into the superhero genre. First, the anti-democratic view of society: In both neoliberalism and superhero movies, politics and big political decisions happen because the elite (politicians or superpeople or supervillains) make them happen. Society is

> ruled over by benevolent philosopher-kings (plutocrats or superheroes or both) who watch over us and aid only when needed; much of the superhero-movie narrative is devoted to litigating the benevolent philosopher-king's specific ideals … Darkest of all, superhero movies posit that humans *need* authority figures – that we cannot survive without policing. It is a troubling moral in an era in which a militarized police force routinely carries out sprees of racist violence on people of colour.
>
> (*op. cit.*)

It's clear this is not just a phenomenon of the Trump era but a phenomenon of this epoch of twenty-first-century capitalism. The global market, the schisms in society, the lack of realistic utopias, the film production process itself, the seemingly endless need for interlinked transnational product and the rise of gaming have all contributed to the superhero film becoming the pre-eminent cinematic genre of the twenty-first century, certainly in terms of box office. Disney look set to expand this dominance to the streaming business, Netflix via shows like *The Umbrella Academy, Sweet Tooth* and *Sandman* are investing heavily in the creation of such 'universes'. The genre has grown for the last 20 years in popularity, and through hybridisation and the co-opting of other genres has morphed and increased its dominance, as Spencer explains:

> The superhero narrative assures us that the world is divisible into simple right and wrong / heroes and villains, and it locates us, via identification, in a place of insuperable power within this world – always on the side of the right and good. But in recent years, the genre has begun to fracture, thus also fracturing the inevitable moral and physical success of the (super)hero through grim tonality (e.g., *The Dark Knight*), the heroes' mortality (e.g., *Avengers: Infinity War*), or simply satire (e.g., *Thor Ragnarok*). This greater complexity has allowed the superhero narrative to develop from genre film to … the 'dominant mode' of contemporary cinema. At the same time, this fracturing makes evident what has been the creeping impact of the superhero narrative all along: namely, that as audiences are encouraged to feel the moral and material righteousness of (their own) power through these figures, the superhero film has a more or less direct connection to the impassioned political bifurcation between 'liberal' left and 'alt' right that so many nations, as well as the entire social media-verse, are currently experiencing. It took *Joker*, though, to make this connection explicit.
>
> (*op. cit.*)

Chaos, Trump and Joker

> I could stand in the middle of 5th Avenue and shoot somebody, and I wouldn't lose any voters, OK? It's, like, incredible.
>
> (*Donald Trump, 2016*)

It was a super-villain movie that inspired the most column inches around a comic book film. Todd Phillips' *Joker* burst into the middle of the Trump presidency with an appeal to rage and anger – in America at least, emotions very readily available on both left and right. Interestingly, this is one of two films of those we have chosen, where the *Rotten Tomatoes* aggregated scores from critics is lower than the aggregated score from other reviewers (68/88), the other being the *Revenant* (78/84).

Writing about *Joker* becomes all the more challenging, due to the numerous controversies around its reception. Part of the process around a film these days is the tweeting, blogging and reviewing that goes on – in the case of *Joker*, its premier at the world's oldest festival – Venice, the dizzying combination of art-house aesthetic and Golden Age of American cinema references (*Taxi Driver* and *King of Comedy* most explicitly), legendary comic book iconography and the current political moment led to the film fuelling a debate like no other.

The furore and passionate arguments around the film have variously been described as,

> an outrage. A scandal. An irresponsible exploitation fantasy. A dangerous provocation. A piece of rabble-rousing incel propaganda. A piece of studio product masquerading as a '70s-style art film. A crime against humanity.
>
> *(Gleiberman and DeBruge, 2019)*

All the same, this is an Oscar- and Venice Biennale-winning film with many hugely positive reviews as well as a large global box office. It is the first 'R rated' movie to earn over a billion dollars at the box office. Whether you like the film or not, what is beyond doubt was that it captured a moment in American history and spoke both to it and of it. Incels, white rage, privilege, anarchy, mental health and inevitably Donald Trump, *Joker* portrayed a character in a world gone mad and a mad man in the midst of it.

> Chaos is the measure of the complexity of the world in relation to the capacities of intellectual reduction. From a different angle, chaos is the measure of the excessive density of the infosphere in relation to the psychosphere.
>
> *(Beradi, 2019b, p. 2)*

Twenty-first century information overload makes for complexity and volume unprecedented in human history – rolling news, social media, a constant cycle of notifications – we are weighed down with facts and counter-facts one tweet at a time. Chaos is easier to manufacture when facts are harder to check, especially when we are either, as in the film *Us*, part of some neoliberal middle-class precariat (Lorusso, 2019) or just unable to meet our financial or other basic needs.

In the 1990s, the so-called 'End of History' (Fukuyama, 1992) and the collapse of the Soviet Union, alongside rapid technological change set in motion a surprising turn of events. The opposite of the end of history in fact. As we surveyed in our opening chapter, the millennium ushered in an age of surveillance capitalism (Zuboff, 2019) allied with systemic financial failure with the banking crisis of 2008. The very same year, the now ubiquitous iPhone made what Berardi calls the infosphere or Global Silicon Valley (Berardi, 2019a) available in your hand, anywhere and at any time. In short, we are now overwhelmed with too much information and too little time. Fact-checking becomes a full-time job, especially when the president "lies so prolifically and with such velocity that *The Washington Post* calculated that he'd made 2140 false or misleading claims during his first year in office" (Kakutani, 2018). In the wake of this and the abject failure of neoliberalism to address the failure of the American Dream for most (offering austerity to the poor and lower middle class instead), right-wing populism / nationalism has been on the rise, most successfully in Brazil, the UK, Poland, Turkey, Hungary and the US. By 2015, as we have outlined, this populism had become a sustained and chaotic attack on Western Democracy.

In her book *Twilight of Democracy*, centre-right commentator Anne Applebaum talks about the new generation of right-wing *clercs* (cf. Benda, 1927), as she calls them (compromised intellectuals who engage in political advocacy), who seem to "enjoy chaos, to promote chaos, as a prelude to imposing a new kind of order". That new order, she suggests, is based in the fact that "given the right conditions any society can turn against democracy". As she puts it:

> the arguments of the old Marxist left – met and mingled with the Christian rights despair about the future of American democracy. Together they produced the restorative nostalgic Make America Great Again rhetoric of Trump.
>
> *(Applebaum, 2020, p. 21)*

As Trump himself said, somewhat presciently given the events of 2020/21, "When the country goes to total hell … then you'll have riots to go back to where we used to be when we were great" (Interview to *Fox News* 2014). It is significant that he chose the Electoral College for the fateful march on the Capitol and the ensuing speech that led to a riot. The Electoral College represents one of the weak points of American Democracy and is part of a system that is unfit for purpose, borne out of the battle over slavery. The "illegal votes" Trump called on to have discounted were the votes of Black and Latino voters in cities like Atlanta. He and his supporters genuinely believed – "they might actually break the system and have power without democracy" (op. cit.).

In some sick way, the events of 6 January 2021 in the Capitol building seem to confirm the fragility of democracy in America. Shots were fired by a mob egged on only minutes earlier by Trump, who told people to march on the Capitol to defend democracy.

> Turn your cameras, please, and show what is really happening out here, because these people are not going to take it any longer, they're not going to take it any longer.
>
> And after this, we're going to walk down, and I'll be there with you. We're going to walk down – (APPLAUSE) – we're going to walk down. Anyone you want, but I think right here, we're going to walk down to the Capitol – (APPLAUSE) – and we're going to cheer on our brave senators and congressmen and women, and we're probably not going to be cheering so much for some of them. (LAUGHTER) Because you'll never take back our country with weakness.
>
> *(Trump's speech before the Capitol riots)*

The deaths of five people in the centre of government that day was perhaps no surprise to the many observers of the administration who could only foresee a tragic end to the Trump presidency, and who may have feared far worse.

Bruce Ackerman's 2001 article 'Anatomy of a Constitutional Coup', which thoroughly contextualises and analyses the American democratic process and Bush's controversial victory over Gore in 2000, is a salutary lesson in the weakness of the federalist Electoral College system. One might say that the 2020 election was the mother of all stress tests – one the system barely passed. As Ackerman describes it, the 2000 Bush / Gore election was effectively stolen when,

> the normal caution was swept aside by the Electoral College. Despite Gore's national lead of half a million votes, Florida's 25 Electoral College votes turned on a few hundred ballots. Suddenly, it made sense for both sides to go for broke. This point was made most explosively in Miami, where more than ten thousand ballots had been rejected by the city's pathetically inadequate voting technology. As the election board prepared for a manual recount, a Republican mob successfully intimidated them into calling it quits. These unforgettable scenes, beamed across the world, will darken the image of American democracy for a long time to come. There is more to these television pictures than meets the eye. Who funded and organised the Republican mob?
>
> *(Ackermann, 2001)*

Nothing has changed with the Electoral College since the debacle and injustice of 2000 because the system requires a two-thirds majority in both houses, along with the presidential will and blessing. The Democrats and the Republicans are locked in deadlock at worst, stasis at best, in both houses, and have been for most of the last 100 years.

Why Is It Always Me? American Exceptionalism and the Joker Trump

Trump's whole *modus operandi* throughout his presidency has been to test this already vulnerable system. He rode to power on the idea of breaking the establishment – the neoliberal elite. He fulfilled this promise in one singular way – presidential protocol was gone with Trump. He said what he liked – usually on Twitter, from which he was finally banned post-Capitol riot, without any recourse to the traditions of his office. He was the trickster, the jester, the meddler. A "breaker" as Snyder describes him and his allies – Steve Bannon, the Breitbarters, QAnon and the Proud Boys, who gathered at his side before the attack on the Capitol:

> When Donald Trump stood before his followers on Jan. 6 and urged them to march on the United States Capitol, he was doing what he had always done. He never took electoral democracy seriously nor accepted the legitimacy of its American version.
>
> Even when he won, in 2016, he insisted that the election was fraudulent – that millions of false votes were cast for his opponent. In 2020, in the knowledge that he was trailing Joseph R. Biden in the polls, he spent months claiming that the presidential election would be rigged and signalling that he would not accept the results if they did not favour him. He wrongly claimed on Election Day that he had won and then steadily hardened his rhetoric: With time, his victory became a historic landslide and the various conspiracies that denied it ever more sophisticated and implausible.
>
> *(Snyder, 2021)*

Trump may not be in the White House anymore, nor even on Twitter, but he still haunts, stalks, you might say, democracy. *Joker*'s end sequence stands now as chronicle of a riot foretold. To use the parlance of the superhero genre, without Trump impeached, and voting rights under assault, an attempted sequel in 2024 now feels inevitable.

Batman's nemesis, the Joker has always been associated with chaos, from his early origins in 1940s DC comics through to Nolan's *The Dark Knight*. A villain whose sole purpose is to sow madness and chaos for no other reason than for the satisfaction of his own insanity. In some ways it was (particularly once Steve Bannon was ousted) Trump's unclear ideology or his narcissistic "ideology of me" that led to his downfall. He wanted to break the system, but like the Joker, more for his own hedonistic ends than through some grand design or ideology.

Joker as Mental Health Comedy

As the Smiths say in their song 'That Joke Isn't Funny Anymore' (1985), "It isn't funny because it is too close to home and too near the bone."

In his depressing and enlightening study of the endemic cults of mass murder and suicide in American society, *Heroes* (2015), Franco Berardi opens with a description of the "very real" attack on a cinema audience by James Holmes. Holmes killed 12 people and injured 70 others in an attack at the Aurora cinema in Colorado. The victims were the audience of *The Dark Knight Rises*. The chapter on this 'phenomenon' goes on to examine Holmes and the culture around him. The chapter is called 'The Joker', a moniker Holmes was given by the media.

In his later work, *The Second Coming* (2019b), Berardi returns to the scene of new but similarly horrifying crimes:

> On 1 October 2017, fifty-eight people were killed and more than 500 injured by a gunman in Las Vegas. As the news spread over the airwaves and on the net, the Fox News anchor-man (and sexual harasser) Bill O'Reilly boiled the massacre down to six words: 'This is the price of freedom.' Oh yes, freedom. Freedom to stockpile weapons, and to order ammo online. Freedom to outfit guns with bump stocks to make them fire faster, as the Vegas shooter did. This is the price of freedom, all right. When a young man called Kelley, just thirty-four days after Vegas, gunned down twenty-six persons during a church service in Sutherland Springs, Texas, President Trump shrugged away the massacre saying that it had nothing to do with guns, only with mental health. Oh yes, mental health. President Trump is an expert on mental health, of course, and a super-expert on mental suffering, as he won the election thanks to the epidemic of depressive rage. The problem is that mentally disturbed people are no longer an innocent minority of the overall population. Mental suffering is more American than Coca-Cola, more American than the stars and stripes.
>
> *(Berardi, 2019b, p. 79)*

In *Joker*, Phillips shows the violence – Fleck kills several people during the film, including the real or imagined murder of his love object, his African American neighbour – but the director is only interested in the surface. I would suggest that the various readings, outrage and praise for the film, lie in the fact that it uses so many references from both real-world events and from comic mythology and from movies themselves that it is open to endless interpretation. Its incoherence makes it such. Is this deliberate or unconscious on the director's part? Muddled thinking or strategy? Should we read more into the use of known paedophile Gary Glitter's music for an iconic sequence?

Incoherence and obfuscation, as Trump has shown, is its own form of chaos – this is what allows such a multitude of readings and at the same time allows Phillips to have it all, without really saying anything definitive. Undoubtedly however, he catches a moment, a vein of American emotion, the anger of a mob, bristling under the surface.

In terms of its overt references to other films, like De Palma ripping the guts out of Hitchcock's *Vertigo* in his 1970s exploitation flick *Dressed to Kill*, there is something tawdry, something exploitative and empty about the homages to Scorsese's *King of Comedy* and *Taxi Driver* in *Joker*. The homage to that New York is empty, a winking nod to a look rather than a serious engagement. In Ramsay's *You Were Never Really Here* (see Chapter. 8), we see how nods and references to other cinema abound but with some purpose; the pleasure of pure cinema gives us a sense of underlining meaning via form and theme.

It's no coincidence that, in the same month that *Joker* was released, Scorsese gave an interview criticising the superhero franchises, which caused such a furore that he followed it up with an op-ed in the *New York Times* (Scorsese, 2019). As he put it,

> So, you might ask, what's my problem? Why not just let superhero films and other franchise films be? The reason is simple. In many places around this country and around the world, franchise films are now your primary choice if you want to see something on the big screen. It's a perilous time in film exhibition, and there are fewer independent theaters than ever. The equation has flipped, and streaming has become the primary delivery system. Still, I don't know a single filmmaker who doesn't want to design films for the big screen, to be projected before audiences in theaters.

Scorsese recognises the superhero film as part of a trend in cinema towards spectacle and away from character and story and theme:

> I developed a sense of movies – of what they were and what they could be – that was as far from the Marvel universe as we on Earth are from Alpha Centauri. For me, for the filmmakers I came to love and respect, for my friends who started making movies around the same time that I did, cinema was about revelation – aesthetic, emotional and spiritual revelation. It was about characters – the complexity of people and their contradictory and sometimes paradoxical natures, the way they can hurt one another and love one another and suddenly come face to face with themselves.
>
> *(Martin Scorsese, 2019)*

In *The Society of the Spectacle* Guy Debord's 1967 work, the author describes a world where passive identification with the spectacle supplants genuine political activity. Debord argues that the spectacle overwrites the past, eliding it with the future into an undifferentiated mass, a type of never-ending present like the anal bolus that Chasseguet-Smirgel (1991) attributes to the pervert; in this way the spectacle prevents individuals from realising that the society of spectacle is just a moment in history, one that could be overturned through revolution.

Phillips himself said he was motivated to make the film because,

> Go try to be funny nowadays with this woke culture …There were articles written about why comedies don't work anymore—I'll tell you why, because all the fucking funny guys are like, 'Fuck this shit, because I don't want to offend you.' It's hard to argue with 30 million people on Twitter. You just can't do it, right? So, you just go, 'I'm out.' I'm out, and you know what? With all my comedies—I think that what comedies in general all have in common—is they're irreverent. So, I go, 'How do I do something irreverent, but fuck comedy? Oh, I know, let's take the comic book movie universe and turn it on its head with this.' And so that's really where that came from.
>
> *(Phillips interview, 2019)*

Director Taika Waititi, among others, called him out for this, but like many, as screenwriter and playwright David Hare (2021) points out,

> When writers from the *Spectator* form a Free Speech Union, its aim is not, as you might hope, to expand the range and quality of public expression by attacking the ruthless no-platforming of non-conformists in the *Daily Mail*, the *Daily Telegraph*, the *Sunday Times*, the *Sun* and the *Times.* Nor is its interest in addressing the covert problems of censorship caused by minorities being under-represented in the mainstream. No, its purpose is to concentrate its efforts exclusively on protecting the right to give offence.

Phillips stands strongly by his right to offend. Similarly, *Joker* sets up its own world – Gotham City – where the tropes of the 1970s New York of Scorsese's lens are set against YouTube clips and comic book asylums. Plot points include violent attacks based loosely in real-life NYC history (some of which like the Central Park Five include and directly incriminate Trump). Like the film itself, Phillips' Gotham bears a multitude of relationships to a variety of times and places in our real world, the cinema of the 1970s and the DC universe, but no real integrated relationship to any one place or time. It's difficult to deal with Fleck's pain and mental health seriously whilst remaining irreverent and operating within comic book mythologies. But as Bainbridge (2021) describes it – "Todd Phillips' Joker has become a popular cultural object that evokes the lived experience of the neoliberal conjuncture, its collapse, and the rise of a new wave of populism."

However, is *Joker* pastiche posturing as mental health tragedy? As Jameson puts it:

> Pastiche is, like parody, the imitation of a peculiar or unique, idiosyncratic style, the wearing of a linguistic mask, speech in a dead language.

> But it is a neutral practice of such mimicry, without any of parody's ulterior motives, amputated of the satiric impulse, devoid of laughter.
>
> *(Jameson, 1998, p. 5)*

Despite, or perhaps because of all these contradictions, the images and the spectacle haunt me still. They arrived empty but in some way were given life and meaning by the riot at the Capitol. As the unorthodox critic, A. S. Hamrah (2018) said:

> The riot scenes near the end of *Joker* reflect something true in society, and they brought the film out of its shell. If you see *Joker*, it would be best to see it in a theater with a potential psychopath for that added thrill of maybe not surviving it. Seeing it at home will be a waste of time unless you live with someone who might kill you while it's on.

Despite its flaws, its mixed messages, its incoherence, the film clearly captures the moment, of post-truth, the mob and of mass deception, strikingly and brilliantly. A spirit of the age. An age where the persistent failure of the American Dream, felt most particularly post-2008 crash, was met by the disruptive breakers of populism. As Sean Redmond put it in his introduction to an issue of the *New Review of Film and Television Studies* devoted to *Joker*:

> Many Americans gravitated to or were seduced by this populism. In the precarious marketplace, tens of millions of people found themselves living below the poverty line, on zero-hour contracts, unable to afford basic food or healthcare. Social support services had been cut and a despairing loneliness had affected all demographics, becoming the crisis of the age. And yet, of course, people had also got (super) rich, the value of the stock-market had risen, and those on the breadline also lined up to celebrate this new Trumpian nationalism. In *Joker* we find these realities, collisions, and intersections played out.
>
> *(Redmond, 2021)*

Trump's exhortation to march on the Capitol and the ensuing riot is written into the DNA of the film. Again, as Hare (2021) says:

> Before Trump, the common pieties of public life had meant that any elector who had sexist or racist feelings, or who wanted always to insist on their own needs over the needs of others, might have felt vaguely rebuked by notions of good and bad. A scent of disapproval would have reached them from the religious and non-religious institutions which were there to suggest social norms. But, under Trump, all bets were off. People of all backgrounds, super-rich and dirt poor, were given permission to feel whatever they damn well pleased by a president who proclaimed, 'Look at me, I'm never ashamed. I'm never contrite. Why should you be?'

The spirit of *Joker* is the spirit of the time. Angry, chaotic, shameless, mob ridden. This is a world where everyone feels hard done by. A world where the most privileged present themselves as 'poor me'. A world where everyone is left out and no one is satisfied. A world where 70 million people vote for a failed president. America – a country openly at war with itself.

References

Ackermann, B. (2001) 'Anatomy of a Constitutional Coup'. *London Review of Books*, 23 (3) (8 Feb).

Applebaum, A. (2020) *Twilight of Democracy: The Failure of Politics and the Parting of Friends*. London: Allen Lane.

Bainbridge, C. (2021) 'Cracking up: Joker and the mediatisation of the arse-end of the world'. *New Review of Film and Television Studies*, 19 (1): 54–64. doi:10.1080/17400309.2020.1861882

Bakhtin, M. M. (1982) *The Dialogic Imagination: Four Essays*. University of Texas.

Benda, J. (1927) *The Treason of the Intellectuals*. Norton.

Beradi, F. (2015) *Heroes: Mass Murder and Suicide*. London: Verso.

Berardi, F. (2019a) *Futurability: The Age of Impotence and the Horizon of Possibility*. London: Verso.

Berardi, F. (2019b) *The Second Coming*. London: Polity.

Chasseguet-Smirgel, J. (1991) 'Sadomasochism in the Perversions: Some Thoughts on the Destruction of Reality'. *Journal of the American Psychoanalytic Association*, 39: 399–415.

Chasseguet-Smirgel, J. (1999) 'The Devil Religion: Some Reflections on the Historical and Social Meanings of the Perversions'. *Journal of Clinical Psychoanalysis*, 8 (3): 381–400.

Debord, G. (1967) *The Society of the Spectacle*. London: Black and Red.

Fairbairn, W. R. D. (1952) *Psychoanalytic Studies of the Personality*. London: RKP.

Fukuyama, F. (1992) *The End of History and the Last Man*. London: Free Press.

Gibbens, B. (2001) 'Professor of English at University of Arkansas at Little Rock,' quoted epigraph in *Napalm and Silly Putty* by George Carlin. Hachette Books.

Gleiberman, O. andDebruge, P. (2019) 'Variety Critics Debate Joker', *Variety*.

Hamrah, A. S. (2018) 'The Earth Dies Streaming', *n + 1*.

Hare, D. (2021) 'Populism without the people'. *New Statesman*, 25 March.

Hassler-Forest, D. (2012) *Capitalist Superheroes*. London: Zero Books.

Jameson, F. (1998) *Postmodernism and Consumer Society in Postmodernism and the Cultural Turn*. London: Verso.

Kafka, F. (1915) *Metamorphosis*, Reprint edition (2009). Martino Fine Books.

Kakutani, M. (2018) *The Death of Truth*. William Collins

Lorusso, S. (2019) 'Entreprecariat: Everyone is an entrepreneur. Nobody is safe. Marcuse, H. (1969) Repressive Tolerance'. In R. Wolff, B. Moore Jr, H. Marcuse (eds.), *A Critique of Pure Tolerance*. Boston: Beaker Press.

Milton, J. (1674) *Paradise Lost*. Book IV. Line 108.

Phillips, T. (2019) Joaquin Phoenix interview. *Vanity Fair*. https://www.vanityfair.com/hollywood/2019/10/joaquin-phoenix-cover-story

Redmond, S. (2021) 'That Joke Isn't Funny Anymore: A Critical Exploration of *Joker*'. *New Review of Film and Television Studies*. https://nrftsjournal.org/white-riot-a-joker-roundtable/

Trump, D. (2016) ‘Speaking at the Sioux centre’, 23 Jan.
Spencer, K. (2018) ‘Peak superhero? Not even close: How one movie genre became the guiding myth of neoliberalism’, *Salon.com*. https://www.salon.com/2018/04/28/how-superhero-films-became-the-guiding-myth-of-neoliberalism/
Scorcese, M. (2019) ‘I Said Marvel Movies Aren’t Cinema. Let Me Explain’. *The New York Times*. https://www.nytimes.com/2019/11/04/opinion/martin-scorsese-marvel.html
Snyder, T. (2021) ‘The American Abyss’. *The New York Times*, 9 Jan.
Vary, A. (2020) ‘Star Wars and Marvel’s futures now flow through Disney Plus’. *Variety*. https://variety.com/2020/tv/news/disney-plus-star-wars-marvel-pixar-series-1234850947/
Zuboff, S. (2019) *The Age of Surveillance Capitalism*. London: Profile Books.

8

YOU WERE NEVER REALLY HERE (RAMSAY, 2017)

Being the Law and PTSD

Internal Worlds

The Moral Defence

According to Fairbairn, as the child grows and develops, and its experience of the world expands, the endopsychic structure develops to become more complex. Initially it is satisfactory relationships that are internalised in the first oral stage. With the eruption of teeth and the ability to direct aggression, in the second oral phase, object relationships can be differentiated into good and bad and internalised as such. As the internalised good and bad relationships threaten to throw the relationship with mother or primary caregiver out of kilter, a need for some further control over their activation is required and a further differentiation of relationships develops. This is based upon those relationships that are acceptable (*Central Self*), those that are over-exciting (*Libidinal Self*), and those that are over-rejecting (*Antilibidinal Self*). The *Central Self* is built around acceptable relationships and strengthened against the demands of other potentially disruptive relationships by the idealisation of aspects of the acceptable relationships that become the basis of an *Ideal Self*.

It is at about this point in the development of the child that Fairbairn introduces the concept of the *Moral Defence*.

> The earliest form of defence resorted to by the developing ego in a desperate attempt to deal with internalised bad objects … repression … the bad objects are simply banished to the unconscious.
>
> *(Fairbairn, 1952, p. 65)*

DOI: 10.4324/9781003206224-9

> I have already spoken of the child 'taking upon himself the burden of badness which appears to reside in his objects' … The bad objects which the child internalises are unconditionally bad … in so far as his ego has a relationship with them, he too is unconditionally bad. To redress this state … he internalises his good objects which thereupon assume a super-ego role … Once … established … we are confronted with conditional badness and conditional goodness.
>
> *(ibid., p. 66)*

That is, good or bad from a *moral* standpoint. Fairbairn suggests that this might be best understood by framing it in religious terms: "it is better to be a sinner in a world ruled by God than to live in a world ruled by the Devil' (p. 66).

In order to stabilise the early relationships between mother and child, the child needs to learn some aspects of the moral codes of the society they are living within. One way is to internalise relationships with the ideal mother into the *Ideal Self* as ego-object dyads, but as Freud pointed out in *On Narcissism*, these relationships can be reversed and used in that form too. If mother is perceived as being cruel to you, you can reckon that she is in the right and her cruelty must be justified, that you indeed deserve to be treated like that. The *Moral Defence* therefore involves the inversion in the eyes of the child of bad behaviour by parents on undeserving children into fully justified behaviour by parents for reprehensible behaviour by children themselves, even if they cannot see or understand what they did wrong.

In *You Were Never Really Here*, Joe's continual need to punish himself, in phantasy at least, his imagining himself killing or harming himself and his flirtation with that real possibility – his knife play and auto asphyxiation – are clear examples of a return of the internalised and repressed bad object relationships breaking the repression barrier and reappearing in his everyday life. And his 'work', which is to rescue abducted and abused underage girls, is clearly restorative / reparative in that it is also a rescue phantasy for himself.

Central Self

The main candidate for the *Central Self* is Joe. But Joe is a deeply disturbed and wounded human being. On the insubstantial evidence of flashbacks, Joe is a veteran of the Gulf War and a former FBI and / or DEA agent working on human trafficking. He is now back home looking after his mother, who is in the early stages of dementia. Based upon these flashbacks, we learn that Joe was abused for years by his violent father, despite his mother's best efforts to protect him. He is deeply scarred, physically and mentally, and has used the *Moral Defence* to excuse his father's hatred of him and taken all of his father's badness into himself to such an extent that his every waking hour is filled with phantasies of killing himself, i.e., the part of himself that is identified with his father. The identification with his father is represented by the ball-peen hammer that is the weapon of choice for both of them. Joe's *Central Self* is beset on all sides by doubts and fears, he is unstable and cannot stand being made to wait, he is a creature of impulses that he curtails obsessively through his preparations for carrying out a job. In order to earn any money, he has become an 'avenging angel' – taking on the quasi-parental task of rescuing young girls from their traffickers and returning them to their parents whilst exercising maximum force on the perpetrators.

Libidinal and Ideal Self

Joe is deeply divided and hidden from himself, clinging to the last vestiges of sanity through his relationship with his mother. He gets a new 'job' from a politician whose daughter has gone missing but who has been told where she is being trafficked. Joe gets her out of this brothel for underage girls and is taking her back to her father when he is attacked by some corrupt cops, trying to get the girl back for the traffickers. We learn from the TV that the girl's father has meanwhile committed suicide.

Joe escapes, killing his captors, and goes in search of the girl. He discovers that, in their attempts to trace him, the cops, and the mobsters who control them, have tortured and killed his contacts with the underworld through whom he used to get his jobs. They have also executed his mother who is, in different aspects, both his (probably preconscious) *Libidinal Self* – they play games together, and share warm feelings for each other, and *Ideal Self* – he cares for her deeply and is gently and humorously looking after her in a long-suffering way, protecting her from harm, and, harming herself.

Joe kills the two mobsters who killed his mother, but also shares the last moments of one of them as they die, in a caring way. He then goes to a wooded lake to inter her body and perhaps kill himself. As her plastic-wrapped body, weighed down with stones, sinks to the bottom of the lake, Joe, who has submerged himself in the lake, imagines he sees the girl he rescued under the water too. An abused child like himself, he is reminded that she is still in need of help. He struggles to the surface of the lake and begins to track down a senator, who is also a mayoral candidate, an *Antilibidinal Self*, who was a friend of the girl's father and is a serial abuser of young girls.

Antilibidinal Selves (Internal Saboteurs)

The original *Antilibidinal Self* who attacked both Joe and his mother, but whom Joe has also internalised to some degree, was his father. All of the abusers of underage girls are *Antilibidinal Selves*, and Joe dispatches them with a ball-peen hammer like the one his father used when Joe, and his mother, were physically abused when he was a child, and he was powerless to do anything about it, other than block out the horror by auto-asphyxiation using the plastic protection that dry-cleaners use for coats and dresses, a practice/defence he still employs when the temptation to kill himself becomes too great.

Libidinal and Antilibidinal Selves

The senator has taken the girl to his mansion on Long Island. When Joe gets into the mansion having killed the guards, he finds the senator in the master bedroom with his throat cut having been killed by the girl who is now, like Joe, both an innocent victim and guilty of murder. This conjunction of good and evil in one person is like the developmental step towards a realistic understanding of others, who are often both, and are simultaneously loved and hated. Joe has a number of flashbacks to earlier traumas, suggesting that there is some degree of integration of these traumas going on.

Joe breaks down and cries; for himself, for the girl, who he finds eating breakfast in the dining room of the mansion, a bloody cutthroat razor by her side. They are now alike in that both have been abused and both have now taken their revenge on the perpetrator. Joe and the girl leave together and go to a diner for a milkshake. In the diner, the girl asks Joe where they are going, and he tells her that she can choose.

In loco parentis

When she goes to the lavatory of the diner, Joe imagines committing suicide again. When she returns, she touches his bowed head gently to wake him. It is like a benediction, and she says that it is a beautiful day. He appears renewed, and they leave the diner.

Perhaps she has found a non-abusive parental figure who will look after her and protect her, and he has found someone vulnerable to love and cherish and protect as he did his mother, as his mother did him, as well as she was able. Perhaps now he can become a father. They might both have become, or have opened the way to becoming, the other's *Ideal Self.* However unlikely, this might be the start of something life-giving for them both.

Throughout the film Joe oscillates between the over-exciting (libidinal) and the over-rejecting (antilibidinal) as he tries to find some stability, some place upon which to ground his *Central Self.* His mother's dementia and death make this very difficult until one of the victims of child abuse, like himself, shows that she is capable of fighting back successfully, and that she trusts Joe deeply. This might allow them both to become more stable and keep the demons at bay as they struggle, restitutionally, to become a loving father-and-daughter-like couple, but this might also just be wishful thinking.

Borderline States

Joe is an almost exemplary case of a borderline personality. Borderline personality is usually the product of child abuse and the consequent dissociation attendant upon that. Fairbairn's theory is regarded as particularly suited for the analysis and treatment of such conditions; it is no great surprise then to find his theory being appropriate to an understanding of Joe.

> Borderline personality organization is characterized by lack of integration of the concept of self and significant others, that is, identity diffusion, a predominance of primitive defensive operations centering around splitting, and maintenance of reality testing. The defensive operations of splitting and its derivatives (projective identification, denial, primitive idealization, omnipotence, omnipotent control, devaluation) have as a basic function to maintain separately the idealized and persecutory internalized object relations derived from the early developmental phases predating object constancy: that is, when aggressively determined internalizations strongly dominate the internal world of object relations, in order to prevent the overwhelming control or destruction of ideal object relations by aggressively infiltrated ones. This primitive constellation of defensive operations centering around splitting thus attempts to protect the capacity to depend on good objects and escape from terrifying aggression … Reality testing … is present in borderline personality organization. It refers to the capacity to differentiate self from nonself, intrapsychic from external stimuli and to maintain empathy with ordinary social criteria of reality, all of which are typically lost in the psychoses, and manifested particularly in hallucinations and delusions … All patients with psychotic personality organization really represent atypical forms of psychosis. Therefore, strictly speaking, psychotic personality organization represents an exclusion criterion for the personality disorders in a clinical sense.
>
> *(Kernberg, 2001)*

Grotstein has described Fairbairn's theory of endopsychic structure as "the unsurpassed metapsychology of child abuse and of multiple personality" (Grotstein, 1991, p. 140), and, "the most apposite paradigm yet proffered for child abuse, child molestation, post-traumatic stress disorder and multiple personality disorder" (Grotstein, 1994a, p. 123).

> Within this Fairbairnian perspective he has stressed the autonomy of the endopsychic structures – '… each structure has its own autonomy, provenance, innocence, will (intentionality), rationale (raison d'etre), birthright, blessing, or curse … [and] … 'I'-ness' (Grotstein, 1994b, p. 183) – and discussed 'the dialectics of endopsychic relationships'. Grotstein

> (1992) has noted, in a discussion of psychoanalytic work with survivors of childhood sexual abuse, that … these patients experience themselves to be discontinuous; each of these apparently disconnected selves lives autonomously and independently of each other and may not even know of one another's existence, yet they seem at the same time to have some unconscious relationship with one another (Grotstein, 1992, p. 71).
>
> *(Finnegan and Clarke, 2012, pp. 65–66)*

There are examples of Joe's borderline states within the film, in particular in flashbacks to episodes of child abuse and auto-asphyxiation, to the Iraqi desert, where he has been shot as a soldier, to finding a lorry full of dead Asian girls and women working as a police or DEA operative, and of his imagining killing himself, all of which arise at times of stress and interrupt his behaviour.

This is also, as has been suggested earlier, the place at which regression to infantile dependence can result in pre-oedipal polymorphous perversity.

External Worlds

Ghosts in the American Dream

> Always present, always ticking. All day long, every few minutes, he'd think, I have to kill myself. But in the mornings and before going to bed, the thinking was more elaborate. He knew it was a waste of time – it was going to have to wait till his mother passed – but he couldn't stop. It was his favourite story. The only one he knew the ending of for sure. The past few weeks it always involved water. His plan of late was to slip into the Hudson at night, during high tide, by the Verrazano. The currents were strong, and he would be taken out to sea. He didn't want anyone to be bothered with the body. Once, when he first got out of the Marines, long before he had gone back to live with his mother, he had nearly done it. He had been processed out of Marine Corps base Quantico and ended up in a motel near Baltimore, drinking by himself for a few days and going to a movie theatre, seeing the same three pictures over and over. Then one night in the motel, he had taken a lot of sleeping pills and wrapped his head in a few layers of black plastic bags, duct-taping them around his neck. *He felt himself diminishing, a shadow around the edges of his mind, and he heard a voice say, it's all right, you can go, you were never really here.*
>
> *(Ames, 2016)*

You Were Never Really Here (YWNRH) won best screenplay at the Cannes Film Festival. Lynne Ramsay's translation of the novel is elliptical, cinematic and brutally beautiful. It's a surprise that Ramsay won for best script, given that her work in general, and more so than ever in *YWNRH*, is a cinema of sound and sensation – a cinema of feeling not speaking. Through close-up and detail of hands, of bodies, of faces, of surfaces, she uses the full array of cinematic techniques to place us wordlessly with our protagonist Joe.

Joaquin Phoenix's outstanding performance as Joe both prefigures and surpasses his turn in *Joker*. Along with Ramsay's masterful direction, superb sound design, allied to Jonny Greenwood's score, makes this one of the best American films of the decade.

A reading of the passage from the source novella above shows us how Ramsay repeatedly and masterfully distils words into image. The novella explains Joe's feeling that he's a ghost, and gives us clear reason why. Ramsay invites us inside Joe's mind via the image or the sound. She explains little, instead evoking the sense of foreboding, of hopelessness and of Joe's wish for death, via a purely visual / aural treatment. The answers in the film are rarely found in dialogue or exposition. Songs, screams and diegetic sound offer more clues than words.

Figuring dissociation

The opening sequence itself is exemplary of the way Ramsay uses *mise-en-scène* to create a dissociative atmosphere and feeling throughout. We start with the title cards – as ever an endless list – Studio Canal, Amazon, Film 4, the BFI, Why Not – Americans, French, British – instructive itself of the complexity and miracle of producing a modern Indie Film even with Joaquin Phoenix as its star – every company a producer, a layer of lawyering, some small or larger piece of money and executive producer notes. Over these cards we hear the sound of a plane landing and a kid counting down and being chastised by a man. We cut then to dust particles via the powerful sound design of a breathless gasp to a close-up of a man (Phoenix as Joe) suffocating himself with a plastic bag. Reminiscent of repeated images from *Insomnia* (Nolan, 2002) and Ramsay's earlier work, we return to this asphyxiation horror throughout the film. This is the powerful visual motif of Joe's desire for death right up until the end of the film. It also reminds me of Glass's fight for breath in *The Revenant*. Male protagonists of this era of cinema are often traumatised, split between a desire to act and a desire to escape the world through death. They are haunted by their pasts – ghosts are everywhere.

From here a quick series of splintered images. This is the antithesis of Cuarón's anamorphic social realism. A series of close-ups. A burning polaroid (a call back to the opening of Nolan's outlier disassociation classic *Memento* (2000)), a Bible as extinguisher, a covered smoke alarm, a bloody toilet bowl (strongly reminiscent of the red overflowing toilet that Harry Caul discovers in the denouement of *The Conversation*), the cleaning of a hammer, a destroyed burner mobile phone chip, gaffer tape, a woman's necklace (with the name Sandy).

It is obvious to contrast *YWNRH* with *Joker* because of Phoenix's star turns in both, but his superior performance aside here, Ramsay's nods to past classics of male paranoia are steeped with meaning and effect rather than the empty exercises in style of Phillips.

Next, we go to a medium shot – we are in a standardised hotel room – it is apparent that a brutal murder or violence has taken place here. This is followed by shots of legs (a young woman's first) including Joe's furtively entering the corridor of this hotel and trying to leave. These are clearly motivated, scanning POV shots. Joe is headed away from the front exit to a back door lit by the neon blue lights of cops at the reception. Under all of this action, Jonny Greenwood's driving 1980s-tinged score quickly becomes an integral part of the DNA of the film. This is the third of Greenwood's scores that are for these films what John Williams was to *Jaws* or *Star Wars* – the other two being P. T. Anderson's *Phantom Thread* (2017) and *There Will be Blood* (2007). The deliberate play and power of image, music and design throughout cannot be underestimated. The fractured world, without establishing shots and with our protagonist's face barely seen here, rhymes with the theme and character of Ramsay's film. Joe as a protagonist is shown in camera for who he is – split and absent – the formal mirrors the thematic.

We get our first real look at our hooded figure Joe as the alarm bell punctuates and stops Greenwood's score and we return to diegetic sound as Joe exits this crummy hotel under a grim overly bright security light. In a back alley, without explanation, he is attacked. He fights back, dispatches his assailant almost effortlessly with a swift headbutt, nonchalantly gets into a cab and utters the first dialogue of the film. "Airport". The streets are alive with diegetic sound. The sign on the taxi door identifies Cincinnati as the town.

Everything in this opening is stripped back to its minimum. We watch Joe / Phoenix's blank tired eyes in the back of the cab as the driver sings to himself and Greenwood's bass and synths act as a backing track to the drivers scat. The black cab driver, now shot in the mirror (another meaningful reference – *Taxi Driver*) then seems to sing the title itself – *You Were Never Really Here* – and the title card appears boldly alongside this. This almost Lynchian other-worldly drive to the airport, lit in an expressionist red, blue and green, underline that we are really in Joe's head – and it's a very disturbing place to live.

We cut then to a close-up of a floor-polishing machine. Cleaning – exactly what Joe has just been doing at the hotel. Then Joe appears, now leaning over a water fountain, a long, dead-eye stare. Joe is absent and yet constantly suspicious. He turns his head from the water, and we cut to see for the first time completely where we are. An airport arrivals area. We can tell it's early – the emptiness, the exhausted young woman, the cleaner. This shot captures our world. In the background, a white female air steward marches, heels clicking, to work, crossing paths with the black man who is polishing the floor.

These two represent the world of American work and racial division. Foregrounded is a young woman, hands across her heart, checked out, exhausted, disassociated perhaps, vulnerable certainly. An external representation of Joe's fears – we will learn he is a protector of young women, albeit a violent, vengeful one. We pan across to the object of the woman's own faraway stare, the now empty water fountain. We cut, as it clicks off and via sound return to Joe, his back to camera, on a pay phone to an answering service. He says, "It's done". To his right a poster reads, 'Miles Above the Clouds' an apt description of his mental state and how he might survive the horror of his 'job'.

We dolly into the now empty pay phone booth (Joe is always moving, he is gone), and our introduction to the film at nearly eight minutes is done. Ramsay's mastery of the form is as different to Cuarón's as can be, but equally powerful, a hypernormalised, fractured, expressionist cinema of disconnection.

The main action throughout is punctuated by flashes of images and horrific sounds from three periods of Joe's splintered life. His time as a DEA agent and the discovery of dead immigrant bodies in the back of a lorry, his time in the Middle East where his good deed led to the death of a child, and thirdly his own childhood, where his wildly abusive hammer-wielding father terrorised him and his mother. All of this is seen in brief, brutal frames – explicitly shown and not told.

Ramsay as Auteur

Death and guilt haunt Ramsay's work. In *We Need to Talk About Kevin* she shows how she has mastered time and space in cinema, as we flip flop across a mother's life, before and after a life-changing event. Ramsay clearly understands the power of trauma. Her main characters are always damaged and disturbed – as well as the mother in *Kevin*, who bears the guilt of her son's murdering actions, in *Morvern Callar*, Samantha Morton plays the eponymous supermarket worker who finds her emancipation out of the trauma of her boyfriend's suicide through escapist sex, drugs and rock and roll, whilst in her feature debut *Ratcatcher*, James is haunted by the drowning of his friend Ryan, whom he feels responsible for. Ramsay has spent her career creating a cinema of guilt and trauma, and *You Were Never Really Here* takes us into the heart of the American nightmare – violent, vengeful, a past of war crimes, of child abuse, of corrupt government power and abandoned impoverished lives.

A Warm Place with No Memory

Joe's inner world is full of suffering, and at the same time his violent vigilante approach to it is no answer to the problem. Joe becomes the law. But it's a world where the law has been violated over and over again to the point of meaninglessness. In Afghanistan, on the border and at home, there is no escape from violence or death. Ghosts, the people "who were never really here" populate Joe's world, the desperate Mexicans (of *Sicario*), the PTSD soldiers (of *First Reformed*), the dispossessed (of *Us*), the abused who become vengeful abusers (of *Joker*), the corrupt body politic (of *Widows*), the ruthless vigilante and ghosts (of *The Revenant*) and the brutal violence of vengeance (of *Once Upon a Time in Hollywood*). Joe's end point resembles hope in so much as the life of the protagonists of *Leave No Trace* and *Nomadland* resemble it. An impossible attempt at life outside of American capitalism.

When Joe comforts another "bad man" he has "put to the sword" (*sic*) with his gun, in their dying moments, he lies down next to him, and the two men hold hands. They listen to and sing along with the 1977 Motown pop song "I've Never Been to Me" by Charlene. We clearly hear the lines during this brilliantly bizarre death sequence. Charlene sings that she has been undressed by kings and she's seen some things a woman isn't supposed to see; that she has been to paradise but that she has never been to me, i.e., herself. Referring both to the predicament of the abused girls and to Joe's childhood but also to the problem of understanding oneself, or indeed, even more so – the problem of the failure of the American Dream and a lack of ontological security. Ostensibly it is a song narrated by someone who has had a wealthy hedonistic lifestyle but has never been self-fulfilled or understood themselves. The song being written as it is for a bored housewife by the narrator, a woman with a lavish lifestyle, admitting that money, power and experience has not led her to a place of understanding. The dream is a horrible nightmare from which death offers some escape, some relief.

Intertextuality also plays a part in earlier scenes. Ramsay's subtext or theme is more likely to be heard in the popular culture of film or song than from her protagonist's dialogue. Joe and his ailing mother watch *Psycho*, and later we hear a scene from Frank Darabont's *The Shawshank Redemption* in which the main character Andy (Tim Robbins) is heard telling his best friend and fellow inmate Red (Morgan Freeman) where he would go to escape. He says he would go to a little place in the Pacific Ocean. "Do you know", he asks, "what the Mexicans say about the Pacific? That it has no memory. So that is where I want to go. *A warm place with no memory.*" This warm place with no memory might also be used to describe the recent growing shadow side of America – the opioid crisis; that has taken Prince, Michael Jackson and more than 100,000 Americans a year.

This is the American Dream Joe has no access to, cut off from himself by childhood trauma, he aches for a warm place with no memory of his past or the horrors he has seen, and that we share with him in disturbing flashbacks. A world where Joe sees his life having little value, other than in saving the lives of those like himself – other young vulnerable children who have been abused. There is no system of care in place, no recourse to state help for these kids, and so Joe becomes his hammer-wielding father to free them and enact a pointless revenge fantasy. Does Joe's narrative fit with QAnon's conspiracy story of a high-powered paedophile ring? In some strange way, yes. But the conspiracy stories that feed left and right in America are borne out of the strangeness of a world where PTSD from the trauma of a precarious life is endemic and where YouTube algorithms lead viewers down a clickbait rabbit hole that unites the alts of left and right in some bastardised version of the alternative hippy new age life and the militaristic paranoia of the Alex Jones cohorts. This dissemination of conspiracies is dissected in the brilliant *New York Time* podcast 'Rabbit Hole' (Roose, 2020).

As we have seen time and time again, most acutely during the pandemic, not even American lives matter that much anymore. In America, the freedom of the individual to possess weapons of mass violence is more important than the rights of the society to law and safety. Joe is by his nature a controversial figure, operating on the wrong side of the law with the right intentions, he is merely a short step away from hurting himself and the innocents he tries to protect. It is Ramsay's cinema of the inside of his head that saves Joe for us, through a cinema of sensation. The idea again (like *First Reformed*) that love (for a woman, of his mother, for the girl he rescues) might save him, that he might reach *a warm place with no memory* – a place outside of the American nightmare.

On the other hand, salvation for the corrupt society he comes from is clearly more than ever out of reach. He is forever on the run, in hiding even – from the world and himself. Another type of nomad – still breathing but the bad feeling remains, it cannot be relieved or expunged in a simplistic outpouring of destructive force, as the film / TV series *The Purge* (2013 / 2018/ 19) pornographically suggests. We are back in that cul-de-sac where violent male revenge is still America's favourite story, it seems.

References

Ames, J. (2016) *You Were Never Really Here*. Pushkin Vertigo.

Fairbairn, W. R. D. (1952) *Psychoanalytic Studies of the Personality*. London: Tavistock.

Finnegan, P. and Clarke, G. (2012) 'Evelyn's PhD in Wellness – A Fairbairnian Understanding of the Therapeutic Relationship with a Woman with Dissociative Identity Disorder.' *ATTACHMENT: New Directions in Psychotherapy and Relational Psychoanalysis*, 6 (March): 50–68.

Grotstein, J. S. (1991) 'Review of *Reshaping the Psychoanalytic Domain: The Work of Melanie Klein, W. R. D. Fairbairn and D. W. Winnicott*, by Judith M. Hughes'. *Psychoanalytic Quarterly*, 60: 136–140.

Grotstein, J. S. (1992) 'Commentary on *Dissociative Processes and Transference-countertransference Paradigms*, by Jody Messler Davies & Mary Gail Frawley'. *Psychoanalytic Dialogues*, 2: 61–76.

Grotstein, J. S. (1994a) 'Endopsychic Structure and the Cartography of the Inner World: Six Endopsychic Characters in Search of an Author'. In J. Grotstein and D. Rinsley (eds.), *Fairbairn and the Origins of Object Relations Theory* (pp. 174–194). New York: Guilford.

Grotstein, J. S. (1994b) 'Notes on Fairbairn's Metapsychology'. In J. Grotstein and D. Rinsley (eds.), *Fairbairn and the Origins of Object Relations Theory* (pp. 112–150). New York: Guilford.

Kernberg, O. F. (2001) 'Borderline Personality Disorder'. *International Encyclopedia of the Social & Behavioral Sciences.*

Roose, K. (2020) 'Rabbit Hole'. *New York Times podcast*. https://www.nytimes.com/column/rabbit-hole

9

WIDOWS (MCQUEEN, 2018)

A Heist on Patriarchy

Internal Worlds

Endopsychic structure

There are a number of candidates in this film for the personification of the different endopsychic structures of Fairbairn's theory, but I am going to start by looking at the most obvious candidate – Veronica (Viola Davis). She is in the opening and closing scenes and central to the whole plot and its development, as wife and widow of Harry Rawlings (Liam Neeson), leader of a gang of career criminals who we witness being ambushed and killed by cops after they have carried out a robbery.

Working through the film sequentially, I am going to treat Veronica as the *Central Self* and suggest that initially Harry would have been her *Ideal Self*, her distress and mourning at Harry's death being the two most convincing clues to their relationship as she construed it. At Harry's funeral it becomes clear that he is to be buried next to their teenage son Marcus (another possible *Ideal Self*), which makes Veronica's tragedy even greater. Damage to the *Ideal* and *Central Selves* leave one vulnerable to the repressed unconscious internal *Libidinal* and *Antilibidinal* forces that you are then less able to resist and repress.

Into Veronica's life looms an external *Antilibidinal Self* in the form of Jamal Manning, the black candidate for the Alderman of the 18th Ward of Chicago, whose campaign money Harry and his gang stole in their last, fatal, heist. Manning threatens Veronica with death and demands that she pay back the two million dollars Harry stole. When she says she knew nothing of her husband's business and she has been left with nothing after his death, Jamal tells her to sell everything she has in order to get the money within a month, otherwise, he will be back.

DOI: 10.4324/9781003206224-10

Harry's chauffeur – Bash – who still drives Veronica around, gives her an envelope containing a key that Harry had entrusted Bash to deliver to Veronica in the event of his death. The key unlocks a safety deposit box in which there is a notebook containing meticulously detailed plans for robberies, all but one of which Harry and the gang have already carried out. The uncompleted robbery is for five million dollars.

Veronica decides that her only option, if she is to get enough money to satisfy Manning, is to carry out this robbery with the help of the wives of the other dead gang members who she hardly knows. When she approaches them, she finds that two of the three women are willing to talk, while the third doesn't return her call. The film has already established by this time, through their mourning for, and burial of, their husbands / partners, that two of the other three wives, Linda and Alice, each from different ethnic and personal backgrounds, are in similar circumstances to Veronica but with less manifest regret at losing their husbands / partners, each of whom dominated them and left them with nothing. All of the women are equally vulnerable and equally hard up.

Having agreed to work together to carry out this robbery, under Veronica's guidance, and using Harry's notebook, each of the women has different tasks to achieve. By various, often ingenious, means, they manage to get all of the things they need to carry out the robbery as planned. A fourth wife, Amanda, who doesn't respond initially, has recently had a new baby boy.

In order to put as much pressure on Veronica as possible, Manning's thugs, led by his brother Jatemme, kill Bash, who was going to be the widow's get-away driver. Veronica goes to see if Amanda might drive for them. When Amanda suspects that Veronica is going to try to carry out a heist, she gives her a dire warning. The baby starts crying, and while Amanda is seeing to him, Veronica, through the behaviour of her dog, accidentally discovers that Harry is alive and being harboured by Amanda, whose baby he fathered. Veronica is shattered by the news and Harry becomes an *Antilibidinal Self / Internal Saboteur* par excellence. In her grief at his betrayal, she remembers clearly the death and burial of her son, who now becomes her *Ideal Self.* We are shown in flashback the part that Harry played in their son's death, unwittingly, but characteristically, selfishly dominating him, and helping to provoke his murder by the police.

The women still need a getaway driver, so Linda enlists the help of Belle, her babysitter, a 'tough cookie' from the Projects. At first Veronica is sceptical, but Belle's firm response calms her and Linda and Alice both accept and trust Belle.

Through guile, courage and good planning they execute the plan, during which they accidentally kill the old Alderman, Tom Mulligan (*Antilibidinal Self*), who challenges them at gunpoint while they are making their escape. In the melee Tom is shot dead, but not before he has wounded Alice. They get the money into the van that Belle is driving, only to find that Jatemme is holding her at gunpoint. He forces them all out onto the pavement and drives away at speed. Unprepared to give up the money, they get another car to chase and ram him, forcing the van to crash head-on into a concrete wall, killing Jatemme (*Antilibidinal Self*) outright.

They transfer the money to the car and drive towards the gang's hideout, stopping on the way to let Linda and Alice out near a hospital entrance, where Linda tells the medics that Alice has been involved in a drive-by shooting and that her name is Jennifer, before disappearing into the night. Belle and Veronica part solemnly, and Veronica goes back to the hideout.

Veronica is unloading the last of the money when Harry appears. They have a heated argument, and she calls him evil. He knocks her down and is taking the money when he decides to kill her, but she anticipates him and shoots him dead. She puts the gun that killed Tom Mulligan in his hand and sets fire to the car they used, before driving off with the money.

Early the following morning, Belle (an alternative *Central Self*) puts a goodly sum of money on a chair in the hairdresser's where she worked, to help the woman who runs it. This hairdresser is being overcharged by Jack (son of Tom) Mulligan for the payments on the salon, as he is also doing for various other phoney start-ups for local black women, which he publicly supports but clandestinely exploits. So, he is also an *Antilibidinal Self.* Belle and her daughter drive off to pastures new with their cut of the heist.

Linda (an alternative *Central Self*) is seen going into the shop, which she had been running previously, with her children; she is clearly going to start off from where she was left by the death of her partner. With the money she got from the heist, she is going to try and make a going concern of the shop for herself and her children.

Some weeks later, Alice (an alternative *Central Self*) now fully recovered, goes into a coffee bar, and sits down. Veronica is sitting in the coffee bar at a different table. They notice each other but Alice's friend arrives, and they don't make direct contact. A school principal arrives and greets Veronica, who tells him quietly that there is a bag of money under the table and that she hopes he will use it to rebuild the school library and name it after her son Marcus.

Alice, who we have seen earlier discussing the possibility of completing her education with the money she now has, leaves and is about to get into her car when Veronica comes out and asks her sincerely how she is and gives her a warm smile of mutual recognition. This warm greeting of one independent woman to another, clearly differentiated from herself and recognised as such, as the overall consequence of their working together to overcome their shared problems and reach their well-defined goals, suggests the achievement of *Mature Dependence* for each of the four women involved in the central action of the film.

Central Self

There are multiple candidates for the *Central Self*, each of whom has a similar story in spite of their different ethnic origins, their different skills and ways of living. They are all female, and at the beginning of the film all in thrall, to some degree or another, to husbands or male partners who are unwilling and unable to share with them, or to allow them any real autonomy and freedom. It is only the gang's overthrow that allows these women a way of overcoming their misfortune and achieving something like their autonomy or *Mature Dependence.*

Three of the women find a way of working together, but they are clear from the start that this is a one-off enterprise, done to redress the bad fortune that had been heaped upon them by their male spouses and by Harry, in particular. Harry, totally selfish, has put himself above everyone and decided to get out while still possible. Earlier, we have seen that Jack hired Harry to steal Manning's campaign funds and scupper his election plans. Jack and Harry would each get half of what he stole, and Jack also helped Harry to fake his own death.

At the end of the film, by working together, three of the wives / partners, of the original (male) gang, have developed into strong independent women with their own lives to lead. Another of the women within their ambit, Belle, by joining forces with them, has also become much more autonomous, and with the money she has garnered is able to live her life as she wants.

The exception to this pattern is Amanda, who had an affair with, and a baby by, Harry. She was aware of what he was doing to the gang, including her husband, and the other women, while she was being looked after by Harry. Her fate isn't discussed, but it might be imagined to be grim, with a young child and no other support to help (both of her recent partners having been killed). She was once part of the in-group by default as a wife of one of the gang, but has placed herself in an out-group through her relationship with Harry.

Antilibidinal Self (Internal Saboteur)

There are several candidates for the *Antilibidinal Self / Internal Saboteur*, including Harry, Tom, Jack, Jamal, Jatemme and the other husbands or partners, Carlos, Florek and Xavy. By the end of the film, undemocratic and corrupt Ward politics, with Jack having been re-elected, is all that survives. The Ward itself, whose boundaries have been redrawn to the disadvantage of the Mulligans, seems to be divided along racial lines – black and white. And the possibility of racial tension and intergroup fighting continues because there is no higher authority to which they can all give allegiance.

Ideal Self

The *Ideal Self* for each of the main women has varied as the plot has developed. As long as she could blind herself to the reality of what he was doing, then Harry was an *Ideal Self* for Veronica. With her reparative gesture of endowing the school library so that it carries the name of her beloved son Marcus, she elevates him to *Ideal Self* status. None of the other women has an external ideal, although they all seem to exist within religious communities, which might provide some sense of the ideal for them. Their mothers, or the mother of their partner, might have been an ideal figure for them, but none of these mothers, as depicted, fulfils that role.

The black Reverend Wheeler, despite his fine words critical of the status quo ("ignorance is the new excellence"), tries to play both sides off against the middle while he garners support for his ministry, but not necessarily the community. "Love thy neighbour as yourself."

Mature Dependence

There are back-to-back scenes, about 1 hour 40 minutes into the film, that illustrate aspects of what I have discussed. Overall, we see several women (*Central Selves*) flourishing through working together pragmatically to achieve greater freedom and personal autonomy, by unconventional and criminal means for sure, but not as a career move so much as to redress the wrongs to which they have been subjected, and to restore the fortunes that they have been cheated out of by their men. They are making reparations / restorations against the bad treatment they have experienced.

In a scene in Harry's hideaway, three of the women are preparing for the robbery. Veronica arrives with the codes to the safe. She urges them to move fast and start thinking like professionals, as this is their first and last job together. She reminds them they have just three days to begin to look and move like a team of men, and one of their advantages is that they are women and that no one will think they have the balls to do such a thing.

This could be seen as the formation of a 'work group' in Bion's term.

> 'Work-group mentality' (Bion, 1961: 173) describes the disposition and dynamics that characterize the life of a group, to the extent that its members are able to manage their shared tensions, anxieties and relationships, in order to function effectively; the outcome is a 'capacity for realistic hard work' (p. 157).
>
> *(French and Simpson, 2010)*

In the scene that follows, we hear Alice speaking up for the first time to her controlling boyfriend David, which reflects the conclusion arrived at earlier when it was argued that the widows (putative *Central Selves*) had all become more deeply integrated personally and had thus moved towards *Mature Dependence*, the ability to see the world more clearly without projection and live purposefully, knowing what they are doing.

Alice asks why they never go to his place, which prompts David to say that he isn't her husband and that their arrangement isn't a marriage; he pays, and she gets a nice life. Alice says she isn't dependent upon him to have a nice life, to which he responds by asking what she would do for money if he ended it right now. Alice is furious at his arrogance in thinking that her life is his to offer, and asserts that it is hers, to be ashamed of, or proud of, to fuck up, or make good. David cuts her off with an irritated comment that he doesn't have time for this right now, as he throws money down onto the table contemptuously and walks out.

Endopsychic structure and psychic growth

What is being argued is that the film depicts a process of psychic growth in the persons of the four women working together to oppose and defeat the antilibidinal forces represented by the exclusively male characters. In order to do this, they have to incorporate and transform aspects of their *Antilibidinal Selves* – their now defunct 'partners' – into themselves and then keep these internalised bad objects under control using their *Central* and *Ideal Selves.*

In Fairbairn's theory, "the chief aim of psychoanalytic treatment is to promote a maximum 'synthesis' of the structures into which the original ego has been split…." (Scharff and Birtles, 1984), p. 83). Fairbairn goes on to argue that, involved in this aim are two further aims:

> (a)a maximum reduction of persisting infantile dependence, and (b) a maximum reduction of that hatred of the libidinal object which … is ultimately responsible for the original splitting of the ego.
>
> *(Ibid., p. 84)*

Early in the film, the women's dependence upon their men and the men's hatred of the women, evinced by their treatment of them, is manifest. By the end of the film, this has all been undone. These women, working together, have flourished and are moving on.

> *it becomes still another aim of psychoanalytic treatment to effect breaches of the closed system which constitutes the patient's inner world, and thus to make this world accessible to the influence of outer reality*
>
> *(Ibid., p. 84, emphasis in original)*

In John Padel's (1991) understanding of growth in Fairbairn's terms, the preconscious *Ideal Self* and the conscious *Central Self* grow from their increasingly sophisticated developed experience of the world, but, as he argues, they also grow by taking aspects of the more ancient, unconscious, *Libidinal* and

Antilibidinal Selves and transforming them consciously into positive and tonic new powers through their struggle with the world, to which they are open, thus weakening the power of the irrational unconscious. Much as these widows adjusted and responded to their new situation by struggling to create and carry through a positive way of transforming their everyday lives but not by emulating their male counterparts and becoming career criminals. All of which took wit, courage, faith, love, and thought. They were able to take aspects of the *Antilibidinal Selves* and repurpose them, to incorporate some of the toughness they learned from their spouses and use it to achieve their own consciously restricted ends.

Mature Dependence and the American Dream

We have argued that these women, the widows of the film's title, have reached a degree of *Mature Dependence.* At first glance this looks somewhat anticlimactic when we consider where they are now. One of the women is running a small retail business, one has gone back to education, another has funded a memorial library in honour of her son and the last of the four has driven off with her daughter to make a new life for herself somewhere away from the Projects. They are however all doing what they have chosen to do for themselves, without pressure from spouses or family and they are all newly confident in their abilities and free from the sorts of projective identifications that marked their lives previously. They are not free, liberated or perfect in any way, but they are free to consider their real options and choose and re-choose the direction they wish to pursue without any unintended consequences of their own (unconscious) making. According to Fairbairn, the stage of *Mature Dependence* is characterised predominantly by an attitude of giving, with accepted and rejected objects exteriorised (Fairbairn, 1952, p. 39). They are free as far as possible from compulsion, either internal or external. I would expect to find that many of the courageous people in the NHS and care homes who have dedicated themselves to caring for others during the Covid pandemic, despite the manifest risks, are also maturely dependent.

The most common example of the American Dream is the idea that any American citizen can become the president of the United States. This would require an open society, one not deeply and fatally distorted by questions of gender, race, colour, religion, wealth, education, class and, as we have seen, these films demonstrate that this is not the case.

External Worlds

Refiguring the Devil in Chicago?

> It's embarrassing to us as a nation .... all over the world they are talking about Chicago. Afghanistan is a safe place by comparison! It's true ... People like

> Johnson (chief of Chicago Police) put criminals and illegal aliens before the citizens of Chicago. And it's a disgrace.
>
> *(Donald Trump, speaking in Chicago, October 2019)*

Requiem for a Chicago Dream

In *Widows*, Steve McQueen transmigrates the original 1980s pulp fiction of three working-class women turned bank robbers in Thatcher's London to Trump's Chicago. The film suffers from its ambition, broadening its canvas whilst shortening its running time, but offers much more than the average American thriller. It splices two genres together to address the problem of the opacity of twenty-first-century capitalism, albeit in a twentieth-century manner. The original 1983 Lynda La Plante TV series (which paved the way for her ground-breaking series *Prime Suspect*) ran at six, 50-minute episodes, whilst McQueen's film is just a third of that. When interviewed in Chicago by Philips (2018), he suggested it could well have been a mini-series. Crime in recent years has found its home on the small screen, with exemplars *True Detective, The Bridge, Broadchurch, Happy Valley, The Killing, Mare of Easttown* and *Fargo* being hits around the world. In this golden age of streaming and boxsets, *Widows* would surely have made a fine addition.

What McQueen and crime specialist screenwriter / novelist Gillian Flynn (*Gone Girl*) layer over the original fantasy revenge heist story is Altman-esque, or even straight out of the John Sayles play book. *Widows* has the ambition of *The Wire* or Altman's *Nixon* critique, in the country music scene, *Nashville* or late Sayles, *Sunshine State* and *Silver City*. These directors and works embrace the communal nature of social life, the idea that the intricacies and connectivity of modern globalised capitalism require a broad canvas populated by an ensemble group of characters. This is Altman's approach to alienation in Los Angeles in *Short Cuts*, of David Chase's analysis of crime, drugs, race and politics in Baltimore in *The Wire*, of P. T. Anderson's dissection of abuse and trauma in the 1970s San Fernando Valley porn industry in *Boogie Nights* or similar territory and place in the late 1990s entertainment sector in *Magnolia*. *Widows* is an ensemble piece, in this tradition, a remarkable break for McQueen following on from the singular stories of *Hunger* and *Shame*, but in many ways with its focus on American racial as well as sexual and class politics, not such a leap from his Oscar-winning *12 Years a Slave*.

Moving way beyond the tepid girl gang territory of *Ocean's 8* and having more in common with the seminal *Set It Off*, *Widows* is a mix of the political and the social across a nexus of complex socio-economic relationships in a very specific time and place. In this case, it's the Chicago of Trump's America – a city riven by race and class conflict and subject to gerrymandering and violent crime. A city McQueen looks at vertically, from City Hall and Super Church to Beauty Salon and Sweat Shop. A city that Trump has always held up as the 'Other', the site of fear, his American nightmare; a place where the devil is a black man with a gun.

Widows opens with the sexual and the racial – a long lingering shot of two movie stars kissing in a stark all-white bed and background. Except as McQueen took pains to point out himself, this is not a normal shot, because Viola Davis is a black woman. This kiss is somehow still taboo in Hollywood. Despite the 1960s, or even the scurrilous rumours that racism is dead (including Sewell, 2021), the world is not as straightforward or emancipated as it seems.

It is no coincidence that McQueen chose Chicago as the city to examine in such detail. The Trump presidency saw a national emergency resurface around race – the slow reveal that there really was a white supremacist (or apologist at best) in the White House. The drawn-out denouement of Trump's presidency, being the 2020 long hot summer of BLM protests followed by unsubstantiated claims (by any metric) of a stolen election and the deaths of five people in the storming of the Capitol on 6 January 2021. (See Chapter 7, *Joker*.)

Bursting at the seams with a psychogeographic view of a little-seen Chicago, *Widows* takes in the connections between criminality, corruption and politics and arguably the defining narrative of the Trump years – racial and sexual politics. Chicago is undoubtedly one of the most racially segregated cities in the world. A startling fact examined most prominently by Ta-Nehisi Coates in his extensive work in *The Atlantic* (2014) and his short film on the Contract Workers Union, which examined the history of racist inflated mortgages in Chicago. Alongside this, Carl Nightingale (2012) in his chapter 'Camouflaging the Colour Line in Chicago', calls the city a "… national clearinghouse for techniques that reengineered these imported devices [of segregation] in ways that sparked movements for racially exclusive neighbourhoods that were unparalleled anywhere else in the colonial world". At the same time, Trump has consistently called out the city, particularly in both of his presidential campaigns. In 2016, he appealed to African American voters like this:

> It is a disaster the way African Americans are living in many cases … and I say it with such a deep felt feeling. What do you have to lose? I'll straighten it out. I'll bring jobs back. We'll get rid of the crime. You'll be able to walk down the street without getting shot. Right now, you walk down the street, you get shot.
>
> *(*Washington Post*, 2016)*

Trump's oft-repeated threat to call in the National Guard to restore order to the city is seen as a dog whistle to the white suburban voter. Trump was trying to ensure they understood that black neighbourhoods are the problem, and he was the candidate of law and order. Despite this, it was in cities like Chicago (and Atlanta) that his 2020 election was lost.

McQueen as auteur

McQueen's directorial approach in *Widows* has formal aspects that draw attention to themselves. The most talked about is the one long unbroken shot on a car bonnet, driving through a South Chicago neighbourhood. Over this strange, seemingly unmotivated point of view shot, we hear, but do not see, the conversation between Farrell's Jack Mulligan and his put-upon assistant / girl-friend Siobhan (the two occupants of this chauffeured vehicle). Like the layers in the film, McQueen starts their dialogue with the sexual and the racial then moves into the political. Outside the car, we see the geographical, the habitat that reveals the segregation and deprivation – politics is everywhere.

At the start of the journey, Mulligan asks Siobhan if she's ever slept with a black man. It's a key tell of his racism and insecurity. All the women in *Widows* are positioned as powerless; any access to power or money they have is clearly mediated through their sexual relationship to men. Whether that's the city trader that Debicki's character (Alice) sleeps with for money, or the old school patriarch politician Duvall, the older Mulligan character, who has a much younger wife and talks to the obviously capable Siobhan as if she's just the nanny or some hired help.

Mid-journey Mulligan begins to rant against the city he's campaigning to represent. He asks rhetorically, doubling down on his racism: "Do you know how many shootings happened in this city last weekend alone? 34! These people are killing each other! This is not where I want to raise my children! Dollar signs and empty promises. Anyone who thinks different is fooling themselves."

Like Trump's various "Chicago is Afghanistan" speeches, the code is clear, the message implicit. Chicago is a failed state, full of black people who want to kill his kids or fuck his girlfriend; he wants to live with the other good white people in the safe suburbs. This diatribe takes place as we move, in a matter of minutes, and blocks, past obvious social deprivation, and arrives quite suddenly in a relatively wealthy area. Significantly, the scene ends at his father's house and campaign headquarters. We later learn this will be the site of the heist itself.

It is these moments that reveal McQueen's immense skill as an auteur. He elevates the genre material, draws attention to it, and in doing so makes us question what we are watching and why. McQueen is often at his best at these moments of self-consciousness. In the critically acclaimed *Lovers Rock* (part of the BBC *Small Axe* series), a brilliant example is when the entire blues party breaks into song, giving a transcendent rendition of Janet Kay's *Silly Games*, McQueen makes a connection with the "blues" culture and represents it in a joyful, life affirming way that he handles movingly.

Widows *as a heist on patriarchy*

Despite all the political intrigue of the election story, *Widows* is still very much a heist movie. It opens with a heist gone wrong and closes with the aftermath of a heist gone right. Everyone in the film is trying to steal somebody's money or power, and this is where McQueen's version of the heist joins Altman's version of the political collective or ensemble film.

Heist movies always look at a gang, a group of men (usually) taking on the bank, the state, the status quo, but *Widows* looks beyond its four central characters, devoting ample screen time to politicians, criminals, businessmen and preachers.

As Robert Niemi (2016, p. 17) notes in the excellent *Cinema of Robert Altman*,

> As for Altman's recurrent themes – isolation, madness, betrayal, deception, deal-making, social climbing, gambling, delusion, failure, death – these rather grim motifs add up to a vision of America as an atomised society of driven, often desperate hustlers, a vision that runs counter to the dominant American Dream ideology that simplistically equates individualism with "freedom" and autonomy.

These themes certainly fit with the largely despicable male characters of *Widows* – corrupt councilmen, deal-making clergy, deluded gambling criminals, deceptive violent husbands, murdering white policemen. Normally, heist movies are also largely about masculinity, but here McQueen's all-female team, the widows, are all stacked against the male, the patriarchal status quo.

As Slowonioski and Leach (2017, p. 18) point out:

> The heist has been used for a remarkable number of purposes .... including entertainment but also depicting the struggles of poor men in a world increasingly dominated by 'big business' and the failure of the American Dream.

As Daryl Lee in *The Heist Film: Stealing with Style* (2014, p. 11) argues: "Heist encodes in story form a particular desire to elude the oppressive or limitations of contemporary mass society ...and provide a critique of the socio-economic order."

Niemi (2016, p. 16) also notes:

> Altman also subverts the bourgeoise subject structurally by deemphasising its centrality to the cinematic narrative ... Altman employs large ensemble casts in multi-plotted ... fashion rather than the traditional hero-protagonist ... a formal tendency that carries strong ideological implications.

These Brechtian stratagems, as defined by Niemi, underpin *Widows*. The ensemble or 'collective' film is a tactic for revelation of the connective tissue in capitalism. It's a strategy against the cognitive dissonance of twenty-first-century capitalism that allows one to type notes guiltlessly on an iPhone which was constructed in questionable conditions in China, whilst drinking coffee from Colombia wearing a £15 T-shirt made by workers who all earn less than minimum wage. McQueen wants you to make the connections and reveal the workings of Chicago's corrupt clock.

The heist and capitalism

The seeming and the being of the system, what modern man (and woman) experiences, is one of the aspects that, following on from Marx, most interested cultural theorists Frederic Jameson and Mark Fisher. The way in which capitalism has disguised itself to 'hide in plain sight', to offer itself up to the world as 'the natural order' of things was pre-eminent in their minds. Clearly, McQueen sets out to reveal just this, through the broad nexus of social relations illustrated in *Widows*. Significantly, as we shall see, both theorists also turned to the Heist movie in their analysis of neoliberalism. Heist movies are nearly always about attacks on the centre of power, on capitalism itself, by groups of men, literally and metaphorically locked out of the system.

In an earlier 1974 essay 'Class and Allegory in Contemporary Mass Culture' (from the collection *Signatures of the Visible*, published in *College English* and initially discussed here in the *Sicario* chapter) Jameson spent a great deal of time on identifying class in modern America. As he said,

> One of the most effective anti-Marxist arguments developed by the rhetoric of liberalism and anticommunism, is the notion of the disappearance of class. The argument is generally conveyed in the form of an empirical observation, but can take a number of different forms, the most important ones for us being either the appeal to the unique development of social life in the United States (so called American exceptionalism) … Nonetheless, in order for genuine class consciousness to be possible, we have to begin to sense the abstract truth of class through the tangible medium of daily life in vivid and experiential ways; and to say that class structure is becoming representable means that we have now gone beyond mere abstract understanding and entered that whole area of personal fantasy, collective storytelling, narrative figurability – which is the domain of culture and no longer that of abstract sociology or economic analysis. To become figurable – that is to say, visible in the first place, accessible to our imaginations – the classes have to be able to become in some sense characters in their own right: this is the sense in which the term allegory in our title is to be taken as a working hypothesis. (ibid., p. 843)

Jameson used *Dog Day Afternoon* in the essay to show how this crucial figuring had become more difficult (even in 1974) as multinational capitalism and globalisation increased. He goes on to analyse class via the workers in the bank, the bank robber himself, his accomplice and in turn the local police lieutenant who "comes to incarnate the very helplessness and impotent agitation of the local power structure"

He concludes:

> the whole allegorical structure of *Dog Day Afternoon* suddenly emerges in the light of day. The FBI agent – now that we have succeeded in identifying what he supersedes – comes to occupy the place of that immense and decentralized power network which marks the present multinational stage of monopoly capitalism. The very absence in his features becomes a sign and an expression of the presence / absence of corporate power in our daily lives, all-shaping and omnipotent and yet rarely accessible in figurable terms, that is to say, in the representable form of individual actors or agents. The FBI man is thus the structural opposite of the secretarial staff of the branch bank: the latter present in all their existential individuality, but inessential and utterly marginalized, the former so depersonalized as to be little more than a marker.
>
> *(ibid., p. 856)*

In short, the marker and representative of latter-day capitalism, the one who foils the attack, becomes an expressionless man in dark glasses. He is unknowable, anonymous, unspeaking.

Figuring capitalism in The Usual Suspects

In *The Usual Suspects*, Verbal Kint suggests that the greatest trick the devil ever pulled was to convince the world that he didn't exist. However, it is to *The Usual Suspects* that we turn to see how the heist movie meets its ultimate end game in a globalised multinational neoliberal world. Released in 1995, it became famous for its 'story within a story' and the mystery of its villain, who is both puppet master and member of the hastily assembled gang that are directed to "take down a score". Kevin Spacey plays Kayzer Söze, or Verbal Kint, as he is known through most of the film. He appears to be a meek thief who is teamed up randomly and suspiciously with a bunch of other crooks in an identity parade – the usual suspects (taking its title from the famous line in *Casablanca*).

The film is structured around a police interview with Kint who is the last surviving member of the gang after their last job went horribly wrong. Kint tells the story of their movements, crimes and activities from the line-up onwards, to a detective, who buys it all. At the end of the film, Kint leaves the interview a free man.

Part of the story he has told is of an arch criminal of legendary status known as Kayser Söze who has been controlling the group. The gang have all been killed whilst doing a job they were compelled to do by Söze himself. In capitalist terms, rather than Robin Hoods, they end up as workers whose lives are clearly and easily expendable.

As Ernest Larsen (2001) puts it:

> The film is concerned to depict Söze's criminality as relentlessly brutal and multinational ... Keyser Söze exemplifies essential traits of this globalization, as he seems to be everywhere and nowhere, to be involved in "global", international traffic, and to rely on political supports on a wide scale.
>
> *(ibid., p. 79)*

Post-police interview, Verbal Kint transforms into Keyser Söze, in a brief moment, as we see the detective interviewer realise, he's been duped, as have we. At the end of the film, having cobbled together a story about the events of the past ten days apparently entirely from the labels and detritus of the interview room's contents – the label on a coffee cup, the wanted notices, the notice board itself – Verbal becomes Söze and disappears.

Some critics rounded on the sleight of hand shown by the filmmakers in its dénouement. Kint's role as an unreliable narrator spinning a yarn from table mats and mugs didn't add up, they argued – it was a conjurer's trick, a cheat on the audience. As Kint tells it, Keyser Söze would kill those who stole from him, and we know early on that all these men had transgressed in this way. If the heist movie is an attack on capitalism, in neoliberalism, Söze stands in for the unfigurable – a capitalism that is everywhere all at once – then the gang pays the price of this attack at his hands. There is no outside capitalism, no hope for escape and no hope for objective truth. As Debord put it in *The Society of the Spectacle* (1967, p. 46) – "The more powerful the class, the more it claims not to exist, and its power is employed above all to enforce this claim."

But that's just the point, as Gelly (2014) explains:

The Usual Suspects questions a global and manipulative narrative instance – an instance whose manipulative nature results from its ramifications in a global world and whose power is so global as to endanger the whole of the narrative as truth-based - unlike what happened, as we saw, in films like *Psycho* or even *Citizen Kane* where the revelation of the true signification of the word "Rosebud" for Kane does not invalidate the whole of the preceding narrative. Put simply, the global narrative manipulation in the film is a sign of the extension of the discourse of the film which is shown to have bearing on the relationship between the falsity of narrative and the concentration of the narrative authority on Kint / Soze as a hidden, "global" narrator.

A warning then that the truth, as well as freedom are at stake in a multinational globalised capitalism. One which we could say we have seen played out in real time in the US in the twenty-first century and taken to an extreme over the last four years.

One thing that precedes Trump's presidency is clearly this "everywhere and nowhere" state of capitalism. There is no inside or out with neoliberalism. In short, Söze is capitalism (un)figured as the ghost that haunts us all, and we do his bidding, whether we like it or not. In a sense, *The Usual Suspect* takes the heist movie to the end of itself, or at least the end of the line, for its attacks on and figuring of capitalism.

> This final appeal returns the film to the issue of invisibility with which it began. You can take it lightly – as a magic trick. Or you could say that the film is issuing a warning about a new invisible Satan abroad in the land. The mystery surrounding Keyser Söze's identity turns out to be coextensive with the mystery of who controls the narrative: we realise that the narration has been unreliable exactly at the point when we discover who Söze is. The strategy of unreliability turns out to be linked to the mythic figure of the trickster, who gleefully uses disguise, lying and the dirtiest of dirty tricks to gain control. The unmasked Söze has demonstrated that the varied configurations or principles of order that have been at stake throughout the movie – the law, the team, masculinity, the family, storytelling itself – have been found wanting, limiting, false or inhibiting.
>
> *(Larsen, 2001, p. 87)*

Söze / Kint represents a form of shape-shifting, ruthless, lying capitalism. Omnipresent and invisible. All powerful and unfigurable. Global, invisible, invincible, cruel.

Whilst *The Usual Suspects* effectively banishes the family from the screen (only Byrne's character has a relationship, and one that is brief and professional), Michael Mann's LA crime neo-noir *Heat*, released the same year, takes the family, and looks at how 'work' and neoliberal capitalism effectively destroy it.

Robert De Niro's Neil McCauley, a brilliant serial thief, dies at the hands of his mirror image, the failed family man cum obsessive cop Vincent Hanna (Al Pacino). The two icons meet once on screen – in the film's most famous scene they discuss their lives. Pacino's Hanna says that his life is a disaster zone. That he has a step-daughter who is really fucked up because her real father is such an asshole. He has a wife who he is passing by on the downslope of his third marriage because he spends all his time chasing guys like McCauley around the block. "That's my life", he confesses.

De Niro's McCauley responds by telling him some advice he got from "a guy", to never let yourself get attached to anything you are not willing to walk out on in 30 seconds flat if you can feel the heat around the corner. Reflecting on their situation, McCauley tells Hanna, "If you are on me and you gotta move when I move, then how do you ever expect to keep a marriage?"

McCauley dies because he transgresses his own rules about attachment. Love here, if not women, children and the family even, is the devil. Comparing McCauley to Richard Sennet's examination of modern man in *The Corrosion of Character – The Personal Consequences of Work in the New Capitalism*, Fisher (2009, p. 32) writes:

> Echoing McCauley's mockery of Hanna in Heat ('How do you expect to keep a marriage?'), Sennett emphasizes the intolerable stresses that these conditions of permanent instability put on family life. The values that family life depends upon –obligation, trustworthiness, commitment – are precisely those which are held to be obsolete in the new capitalism.

As Larsen (2001, p. 61) puts it:

> Heist movies are almost by definition intense depictions of men involved in a criminalised work process. In a sense, the heist film both redeems and represses the labour process by representing it as an all-or-nothing one-time venture.

If *The Usual Suspects* is the natural end point for figuring the unfigurable devil of capitalism in the heist movie, then *Heat* is the end of the family in the face of neoliberal alienation. The professional criminals in *The Usual Suspects* have been played, manipulated and destroyed by the invisible devil of capitalism. The police and criminal do what they do because that's all they know – law enforcer and criminal – the recognition is there but the difference is meaningless. In *Heat*, in the midst of all this comes Waingro, a different kind of devil. The crossing point between the cop and the professional criminal – Waingro is the fly in Macauley's ointment, the masculine that truly lives by Macauley's rules. He is a man literally with no relationships – and in that way he is of course completely psychotic. These are the alternatives for masculinity in capitalism it appears. The psychotic Waingro, the violent invisible devil Söze, the working man with tenuous familial ties – Macauley and Hanna.

As Verbal tells it, Keyser Söze would kill those who stole from him, and we know early on that all the usual suspects had transgressed in this way – there is no honour amongst these thieves. If the heist movie is an attack on capitalism, and Söze stands in for the unfigurable – a global capitalism that is everywhere all at once – then the gang pays the price at his / its hands, in the same way Macauley has to die. There is no outside capitalism, no hope for redemption or escape.

Set It Off – What's the Protocol When You've Got a Fucking Gun to Your Head?

Set It Off, released the same year as the *Usual Suspects*, offers a different avenue – one of the few heist movies to feature an all-female gang. *Set It Off* offers an alternative vison of the world, what Mark Kermode (2020) calls "the strange case of *Set It Off*" , it's clearly an outlier moment in the genre and a strong influence on *Widows.* Like *Widows,* it concerns itself with place and time. The four working-class female protagonists are fully based in South Central Los Angeles in 1996. A South Central of racial tension, poverty and little hope – post-1992 riots and post-Rodney King. The four protagonists have little real chance to escape their circumstances, they are not professional criminals but merely office cleaners.

At the opening of the film, one loses her job as a bank teller for not following protocol, when one of the men she knows from her 'hood' robs the bank. By the end, in what is clearly the message of the film, she puts a gun to the pursuant white cop – an unreconstructed faux sympathetic version of Harvey Keitel's conflicted character in *Thelma and Louise* – and asks him, "what is the protocol when you've got a fucking gun to your head?" These four women clearly have the proverbial gun of economic and environmental pressure very much at their heads. They are, as Kermode puts it, "fully developed characters rooted in day-to-day reality." Much like *Widows,* it's a film about "cooperation and loss". Unlike *Widows,* it benefits from using these four women as the pure lens of the story, focusing singularly in on who they are and how they bond.

A World of Widows

In *Widows* the four women, as we've seen in the Internal Worlds analysis above, all have their own American Dreams, all have terrible or no relationships. The values that Fisher (2009) talks about – obligation, trustworthiness, commitment – which family life depends upon, are all clearly absent. The only familial relationships portrayed are abusive parents and controlling, scheming men. The family is dead. The only way out for them is the heist. Like *Set It Off,* for these women there really is no alternative.

Is *Widows* a "turnout-lowering movie", as Richard Brody (2018) puts it in *The New Yorker,* because it portrays everyone on every side of the political fence as corrupt? Or is it an old-fashioned cobbling together of two types of film – the heist and the ensemble film – that would be better served on a streamer over ten episodes that could give McQueen the space for depth of character as well as the juice of the heist and the multiple layers of the city? Time and the development of character is clearly a problem – as Brody (2018) puts it in his scathing review: "The problem is that the movie never bothers to make clear who, in fact, the widows are."

I'd agree that depth of character is the Achilles heel of *Widows.* Despite these problems of overpacking its running time and stretching the audience's credulity at times, it is simultaneously an attempt at something inventive and more radical than many heist movies. It identifies that beyond mid-1990s classics *Set It Off, Heat* and *The Usual Suspects,* the heist movie still has something to say, particularly about patriarchy but also about race.

Widows is the heist movie as an attack on power, from an avowedly female perspective. A film that identifies capitalism not only as a complex nexus of social relations mediated by money without morals but as an intimate bedfellow of patriarchy, of unbridled male power at every layer of society. A world in which men cannot be relied upon as husbands, fathers, or business partners. An unpacking of patriarchy as the bedrock of capitalism.

As a clear attack on patriarchy, does it offer some radical hope? In the denouement, Veronica gives her share of the heist money to education for a library named after her dead son – killed by a policeman on a routine stop, in another of the story's unwieldy but relevant complications. She seems to have no worry about the stolen money being traced, or repercussions for her and her accomplices, which smacks of an unreality that is truly hard to believe and one of the central problems with the film. The film suffers from this suspension of disbelief over and over again, a stretching of credulity even within the bounds of the genre(s) and against a backdrop that conversely takes great care with the authenticity and realism of the city. It is a lack of time and a surfeit of plot that leaves character wanting, I would argue, despite McQueen's bravura direction of the film's many violent set pieces and its quieter emotional moments.

Do the limits of our utopian imagination that Fisher, Žižek and Jameson railed about – the idea that it is easier to imagine "the end of the world than a world without capitalism" mean that only endings like those found in *The Usual Suspects* and maybe, even more appropriately, the glorious nether-world smiling death in feminist road movie *Thelma and Louise* are possible? Has the present moment, the lack of alternatives, strangled our cultural imagination to the extent that even in our wildest dream these widows could not possibly survive against the forces pitted against them – the various worlds of bad men (criminals, husbands, police, politicians, pastors) – or is the title itself the giveaway? That only a world without men in power, or alive even, a world of literal widows, is one where real emancipatory politics might still be realistic or possible? Something like Solanas's infamous SCUM manifesto perhaps?

And if Trump's take on Chicago – characterising it as the devil's playground – doesn't hold water, what will or can Biden do about the failure of not just Trump, but many presidents before, to address the very real and urgent problems of housing, segregation, health and education in America's major cities? What material difference did previous presidents make? Trump may have vilified Chicago and used it for his own racist diatribes, but he didn't invent it. If the GOP is now a battle between the 'gamers' (McConnell) and the 'breakers' (Trump, Cruz, Hawley) what will the Democrat 'status quo-ers' (Biden, Clinton, Obama) now in power, do to demonstrate to those on the left (AOC, Bernie Sanders, Warren) that meaningful change is possible for ordinary Americans? How will they actualise that? Certainly, nowhere will that question be asked more urgently than by women on the streets of South Chicago.

References

Bion, W. R. (1961) *Experiences in Groups and Other Papers.* London: Tavistock Publications.

Brody, R. (2018) '*Widows* Reviewed: Steve McQueen Grafts Politics onto a Heist Film'. *The New Yorker,* Nov. https://www.newyorker.com/culture/the-front-row/widows-reviewed-steve-mcqueen-grafts-heist-film

Coates, T-N. (2014) 'The Case for Reparations'. *The Atlantic*, June.

Debord, G. (1967) *The Society of the Spectacle* (New Edition 1994). London: Rebel Press.

Fairbairn, W.R.D. (1952) *Psychoanalytic Studies of the Personality.* London: RKP.

Fisher, M. (2009) *Capitalist Realism: Is There No Alternative?* London: Zero Books.

French, R. B., Simpson, P. (2010) 'The "work group": Redressing the balance in Bion's Experiences in Groups'. *Human Relations* 63 (12): 1859–1878.

Gelly, C. (2014) 'The Usual Suspects or the potency of falsity'. *Mise en point.* https://journals.openedition.org/map/1646?lang=en.

Goffman, E. (1959) *The Presentation of Self in Everyday Life.* Doubleday: Scotland.

Grandin, G. and Gourevitch, A. (2014) 'Capitalism and Slavery – An Interview with Greg Grandin'. *Jacobin.* https://www.jacobinmag.com/2014/08/capitalism-and-slavery-an-interview-with-greg-grandin/

Guardian Staff Agencies (2019) 'Trump calls Chicago "embarrassing to nation" during first visit as president', *The Guardian*, 29 Oct.

Hanich, J. (2020) 'On Pros and Cons and Bills and Gates – The Heist Film as Pleasure'. *Film Philosophy, 24* (3).

Jameson, F. (1977) 'Class and Allegory in Contemporary Mass Culture: Dog Day Afternoon as a Political Film '. *College English.* April. https://www.jstor.org/stable/375957.

Jameson, F. (1991) *Postmodernism or the Cultural Logic of Late Capitalism.* London: Duke University Press.

Kermode, M. (2020) 'Mark Kermode's Secrets of Cinema, The Heist Movie', *BBC iPlayer.*

Larsen, E. (2001) *The Usual Suspects.* London: BFI Film Classics.

Lee, D. (2014) *Intro to The Heist Film: Stealing with Style.* London: Wallflower Press.

Niemi, R. *(2016) The Cinema of Robert Altman.* London: Columbia University Press.

Nightingale, C. (2012) *Segregation – A Global History of Divided Cities.* London: Chicago University Press.

Padel, J. (1991) 'Fairbairn's thought on the relationship of inner and outer worlds'. *Free Associations*, 24: 589–616.

Philips, M. (2018) 'Viola Davis, Gillian Flynn and Steve McQueen enter Chicago underworld with "Widows"'. *Chicago Tribune*, 8 Nov.

Scharff, D. E. and Birtles, E. (1994) *From Instinct to Self: Selected Papers of W.R.D. Fairbairn. Vol. 1 Clinical and Theoretical Papers.* London: Jason Aronson Inc.

Sewell, T. (2021) *Commission on Race and Ethnic Disparities.* UK Government. https://assets.publishing.service.gov.uk/government/uploads/system/uploads/attachment_data/file/974507/20210331_-_CRED_Report_-_FINAL_-_Web_Accessible.pdf

Slowonioski, J. and Leach, J. (2017) *The Best Laid Plans: Interrogating the Heist Film.* London: Wayne State University Press.

Snyder, T. (2021) 'The American Abyss'. *The New York Times*, Jan. https://www.nytimes.com/2021/01/09/magazine/trump-coup.html

Solanos, V. (2004) *The SCUM Manifesto.* London: Verso.

Trump, D. (2016) 'Donald Trump to African American and Hispanic voters: "What do you have to lose?"'. *Washington Post*, 22 Aug. https://www.washingtonpost.com/news/post-politics/wp/2016/08/22/donald-trump-to-african-american-and-hispanic-voters-what-do-you-have-to-lose/

10

US (PEELE, 2019)

Underclass! The Return of the Repressed

Internal Worlds

Us *as allegory*

An allegory is

> … a story, play, poem, picture, or other work in which the characters and events represent particular qualities or ideas that relate to morals, religion, or politics.
>
> (Cambridge English Dictionary)

Us is a multilayered allegory about modern America, riven from top to bottom by the differences between the 'haves', who are very visible, and the 'have nots', who are invisible. We are talking about a borderline that separates families and individuals – families that are split between those that have wealth and opportunity and those that have no access to wealth or opportunity; and about individuals who are split, between those that have some chance of reaching a productive maturity and those that are tied to self-defeating, self-harming and essentially unproductive activities, with unsatisfied needs and undeveloped powers. Using Klein's terms, people who have reached the depressive position versus those stuck in the paranoid schizoid position, unable to develop any further. In Fairbairn's terms, those who have developed *a basic endopsychic structure and the possibility of Mature Dependence* and those who remain *at the transitional stage or the earlier stage of infantile dependence.*

At the beginning of the film the following is displayed:

DOI: 10.4324/9781003206224-11

> There are thousands of miles of tunnels beneath the continental United States ...
>
> Abandoned subway systems, unused service routes, and deserted mine shafts ...
>
> Many have no known purpose at all.

This reference to the huge area of abandoned underground tunnels in the epigraph at the start of the film conjures an alternative 'Morlock' zone (Wells, 2005), an unconscious, a repressed enclave, from which will emerge the 'tethered', those with extremely limited horizons, the enslaved, all of whom are the product of earlier attempts to control society. This might also be a reference to the so-called 'Underground Railroad', described by the *National Geographic* as "a network of routes, places, and people that helped enslaved people in the American South escape to the North."

While Jordan Peele doesn't use the easy equations of enslaved blacks versus white oppressors, nevertheless there is something of this underlying conflict that informs the film. In a recent short film, part of a Black History Month appraising and contextualising Jordan Peele's work, Ellen Jones says:

> Peele layers political and social meanings ... The relationship between those living happy lives up on the surface and their doubles struggling underground is an intentionally elastic metaphor. Do the tethered represent the world's poor left behind by prosperity, the colonial crimes we'd rather keep buried in the past, or our traumatised former selves?
>
> *(Jones, E., 2020)*

'Find yourself'

The point where the upper and lower worlds meet in the film is a fun park on Santa Cruz beach through a sideshow attraction. Originally, Adelaide is attracted by, and goes into, a Native American 'Vision Quest: Find Yourself' entrance, to a Ghost Train / Mirror Maze, type of sideshow. Thirty years later, when her son Jason sees the same sideshow, it has been renamed as 'Merlin's Forest' but is otherwise the same. The underlying injunction is still 'Find Yourself', but the implied means and the mythologies have changed over the years.

There is no doubt who the *Central Self* of this movie would be, but that self is itself split, doubled, as we shall see, in a doubling that runs throughout the film.

Who is 'us|Us|US'? Is it the family, as when Jason identifies the persecutory family of doppelgangers, and facing them, in a moment of recognition, states, 'They are us!' Or is it the conjunction of Adelaide and Red and their subterranean meeting in the mirror maze (preconscious) between the (conscious) surface and the (unconscious) underground, with Adelaide being forced by Red into swapping places as children? They are both changelings. Each child a product of nature and nurture, each child traumatised. Or is it the US, a country divided by differences in terms of race, gender, education, class and wealth; black and white, rich and poor, male and female, educated and uneducated, employed and unemployed?

The tethered

The ‘Hands Across America’ charity event of 1986, organised to help the poor and needy in the US, which failed to achieve any of its aims (Bailey, 2019) is later rehearsed as a ‘return of the repressed’ underclass, emerging from their underground bunkers to murder and replace the ordinary citizens to whom they are ‘tethered’. There is a telling comment by the organiser of the Hands Across America event, Ken Kragin, who said, “Hands Across America turned our eyes inward”, a view which seems to have been taken up by Jordan Peele alone.

But what does it mean to be ‘tethered’? Normally, to be tethered is to be on a leash, to have restricted movement and opportunities, to be enslaved. A tether is “a rope, chain, or the like, by which an animal is fastened to a fixed object so as to limit its range of movement” (Dictionary.com).

While the pledge on a plaque on the Statue of Liberty boasts: “Give me your tired, your poor, / Your huddled masses yearning to breathe free. / The wretched refuse of your teeming shore. Send these, the homeless, tempest-tost to me, / I lift my lamp beside the golden door!” The reality for the tethered has remained unchanged ever since this was first added to the Statue of Liberty in the early 1900s.

From a Fairbairnian perspective, this story is about a child (Adelaide) who is taken away from her natural family and put into a subterranean society that does little if anything to help her develop her powers further. But she has had a good start in life and has already developed powers of her own. However, she is resentful about her conditions and aware of what the child to whom she is ‘tethered’ will be encountering in the above-ground reality she came from.

The tethered child (Red) also has problems when she is welcomed back by the grateful parents, who mistake her for their natural child (Adelaide). The above-ground parents are concerned about what trauma could have befallen her (Adelaide (Red)), for her to have become so diminished by the experience. In trying to understand her trauma, they talk about post-traumatic stress disorder (PTSD). The differences between the ‘surface’ people and the ‘underground’ people may best be described as the difference between a free people and an enslaved people, traumatised to the point of idiocy and incompetence. The facts that give the lie to all this are that both girls are capable, in the right circumstances, of developing, or regressing, relative to their environmental affordances.

In a strong parallel to those cases of actual abuse and trauma, where the child becomes split in order to defend themselves against the painful realities it cannot avoid, here the child is already two children, albeit connected by a 'tether', according to Red (Adelaide), the exemplary victim of the trauma. As with the investigation of Dissociative Identity Disorder (DID) (Multiple Personality Disorder (MPD)) it is only when the full story can be rediscovered and articulated consciously by the one who suffered it that the reality of what happened can be appreciated. Red was originally one of those in the underground with sufficient initiative to attempt to leave, and sufficient intelligence to formulate and execute a plan of escape, and as a consequence she replaced Adelaide and became Adelaide (Red).

Adelaide was originally in the surface reality, but her curiosity led her to explore the underworld, and as a consequence she was captured and consigned to the underworld as Red (Adelaide). Red (Adelaide) it was that both fulminated against what had happened to her, and so resented it, that she spent years formulating a plan to enable the 'tethered' to escape and take over the US. It seems that it was only in early adolescence when both Adelaide and Red were becoming proficient as dancers, that Red (Adelaide) discovered a religious faith and was able to develop her plans to escape to the surface, and the tethered were able to understand and take notice of her ideas and work with her as a leader, to develop the plan to escape and emerge into the light.

Above ground, now grown up and married with two children, Adelaide (Red) has all sorts of forebodings and discomfort when they go on a family holiday to Santa Cruz beach, the site of the original replacement by her doppelganger, but, like many victims of child abuse, she doesn't remember what actually happened.

A Jeremiad

> I find myself, not for the first time, in the position of a kind of Jeremiah.
>
> *(Baldwin, 1965)*

Red's (Adelaide)'s religious conversion and her plan for the liberation of the tethered are noted obliquely in the biblical references to Jeremiah 11.11 that appear throughout the film, both above and below ground.

> Therefore, thus saith the LORD, Behold, I will bring evil upon them, which they shall not be able to escape; and though they shall cry unto me, I will not hearken unto them.
>
> *(King James Bible)*

This threatened retribution suggests that the early tethered were indeed slaves, who were supposed to be cared for by their masters when slavery was abolished. But the masters reneged on the promise to abolish slavery for the tethered and never made good on their promise. That promise is echoed on the plaque in the Statue of Liberty. As Kimberly Jones, commenting upon recent Black Lives Matter demonstrations said, "They are lucky that what black people are looking for is equality and not revenge" (Jones, K., 2020).

Red's story

It is Red's (Adelaide)'s account that allows us to make sense of the action, while Adelaide (Red) fights to defend and preserve her (adopted) family and her amnesia. The murderous emergence of the tethered above ground is a consequence of Red (Adelaide) showing the same fighting spirit on behalf of her (adopted) people.

While 'Hands Across America' was a, supposedly, benign and charitable attempt to redress the scandalous imbalances within American society, the richest country in the world, it led to malnutrition, homelessness and poverty, and made the American Dream an impossibility for most Americans. The revised 'Hands Across America' is a revolt by those who are oppressed against the society that oppresses them. It is an attempt by the underclass to remake, to liberate, America. To make the American Dream a reality. The example of 'Hands Across America' in 1986 was more or less the last thing that Adelaide, as a little girl, saw on TV before she was kidnapped and exchanged to become Red (Adelaide). Her plan, following her religious conversion, is to transform the 'Hands Across America' approach to uniting the country for charitable purposes, to allow the tethered to escape their subterranean imprisonment, and take over the society that has systematically abused them and kept them in poverty and ignorance.

Red (Adelaide) gives an account of her experience as Adelaide's shadow in the form of a fairy tale. She says that once upon a time there was a girl who had a shadow and the two were connected, tethered together. When the girl ate, she was given warm and tasty food but when the shadow ate, she had to eat rabbit, raw and bloody. At Christmas the girl received wonderful soft and cuddly toys, while the shadow received sharp and cold toys that cut her fingers when she played with them. The girl met a handsome prince and fell in love, while the shadow met Abraham, and it didn't matter if she loved him or not as he was tethered to the girl's prince anyway. The girl had a beautiful baby girl, but the shadow gave birth to a monster. The girl's second child, a boy this time, was by caesarean section, which the shadow had to perform on herself. The shadow hated the girl so much, until one day the shadow realised, she was being tested by God.

When asked who they are, Red's (Adelaide's) response to the question is that they are Americans. And her response to the question of what they want is: that they want to take their time; that they have been waiting for this day for so very long, and they call it the untethering.

Red (Adelaide) explains what has happened first by marvelling at how it must have been to grow up with the sun, the wind, the trees and how Adelaide (Red's) people took it for granted. "It was your people that built it," she says.

> They figured out how to make a copy of the body but not the soul. The soul remains one shared by two. They created a third so they could use them to control the ones above like puppets. But they failed and they abandoned the tethered for generations who, without direction, went mad and then there was US, remember? We were born special.

Red relates how she never stopped thinking about her shadow and how things could have been if she had taken Red with her. Years later, a miracle happened and Red saw God, who showed her the path and that:

> you, the shadow, saw it too and it was the end of our dance. The tethered saw that I was different and that I would deliver them from this misery. I found my faith and began to prepare. It took years to plan, everything had to be perfect. I didn't just need to kill you I needed to make a statement that the whole world would see. It is our time now up there and to think if it wasn't for you, I would never have danced at all.

Post-traumatic stress disorder (PTSD) and the self

When discussing an appropriate therapeutic for the PTSD that Adelaide (Red) appears to be suffering, the recommendation of the psychologists advising on her recovery is for her to be encouraged to tell her story in whatever expressive forms are available to her. In parallel Red (Adelaide) achieves her personal liberation below ground through dance in adolescence. The ability to articulate and communicate her story through expressive dance is the precursor to her emergence as the charismatic leader of a revolution. A revolution that would untether all of the people. In the language of Red's vision, "the soul is one shared by two", a schizoid being that might be transformed from two to one, if one of the two were eliminated or overcome. But in her plan the ones that are to be eliminated are the ones with the technical and intellectual know how, and those that are intended to survive are the least prepared technically but the most coordinated practically. The classic opposition in a revolution between an avant-garde and the workers and peasants. It is the instinctive solidarity of the underground people that might see them triumph, but they will have to invent a new civil and political society to embody and sustain solidarity over individual advantage. Given the relative lack of development of the underground people and their being much closer to being simple bodily egos than selves, some set of unifying feelings and responses would have to be developed within a well-ordered and egalitarian framework to help them survive. Or would such feelings and responses be precisely that well-ordered and egalitarian framework? It would imply something as necessary as, an instinct for relatedness and reciprocity.

It might be useful to take Red's (Adelaide)'s description of their condition – "the soul remains one shared by two" – of what we might call the 'triune (three-in-one) tethered self' and compare it with some well-known psychoanalytic models of the self.

Freud's structural model is based upon three entities – the Superego, the Ego and the Id. If we argue that the Superego is most likely to be identified with the soul, then the overground people could be identified with the Ego and the underground people the Id.

If we adopt Klein's division between the depressive position and the paranoid-schizoid position, then we might associate the overground people with the depressive position and the underground people with the paranoid-schizoid position.

If we use Winnicott's concept of true and false selves, we are likely to conclude that the overground people are true selves and the underground people are false selves.

In Freudian terms, this revolt of the underclass (tethered) is the return of the repressed, but without an extant ego.

In the Kleinian schema, this would be the paranoid-schizoid position without relief, and if the Winnicottian assumption is that the overground people are the true selves, then all we are left with is false selves.

By contrast, if we use Fairbairn's model of endopsychic structure, the soul could be the *Ideal Self*, and the *Central Self* could be the overground people, while the underground people could be the *Libidinal and Antilibidinal Selves* – dissociated, transgressive, possible selves that together represent the ongoing conflict involved in approaching *Mature Dependence.*

I doubt that Jordan Peele had a psychoanalytic conception of these different selves when he made the film (although the Christian trinity and the resurrection of the dead may be implicated in the symbolism of the film), but in a literal sense this is a story of the world turned upside down, one version of the 'Rapture'. It has within it the sort of justified anger of the 'Black Lives Matter' movement.

The Schreber Case and Red's (Adelaide's) attempt to heal the early splitting

Daniel Paul Schreber was a German judge who suffered from three distinct mental illnesses, the second of which he described in his book *Memoirs of My Nervous Illness* (1903) which was used by Freud to understand paranoia. Fairbairn published his thoughts on Schreber (Fairbairn, 1994) when a new translation of Schreber's book appeared:

> Fairbairn takes the position that the pathology involves the disposal of aggression as much as sexuality … and takes into account Klein's

> postulation of multiple internal part objects which disintegrate into a host of internal persecutors projected into the external world … Fairbairn describes paranoia as a way of handling object relations through anal phase techniques, which employ the bodily process of defecation as a model for the disposal of the aggressive projection of bad internal objects.
>
> *(Scharff and Birtles, 1994, p. 8)*

In the Appendix to Melanie Klein's most widely read journal article (Klein, 1946), the author discusses Freud's understanding of Schreber's delusion of the destruction of the world in terms which echo the plan developed by Red (Adelaide) to liberate the tethered and destroy the above-ground people who she feels have deserted her.

> Regarding the processes which are at the bottom of the paranoiac world catastrophe, Freud arrived at the following conclusions: 'The patient has withdrawn from the persons in his environment and from the external world generally the libidinal cathexis which he has hitherto directed on to them. Thus, all things have become indifferent and irrelevant to him, and have to be explained by means of a secondary rationalization as being "miracled up, cursory contraptions". The end of the world is the projection of this internal catastrophe; for his subjective world has come to an end since he has withdrawn his love from it' (Freud, 1911, pp. 456–457) … a little further on (pp. 461–462) Freud considered another aspect of these disturbances. He said: 'We can no more dismiss the possibility that disturbances of the libido may react upon the egoistic cathexes than we can overlook the *converse possibility* – namely, that a *secondary or induced disturbance of the libidinal processes may result from abnormal changes in the ego. Indeed, it is probable that processes of this kind constitute the distinctive characteristic of psychoses*'. It is particularly the possibility expressed in the last two sentences which provides the link between Freud's explanation of the world catastrophe and my hypothesis. 'Abnormal changes in the ego' derive, as I have suggested in this paper, from excessive splitting processes in early infancy … The mechanism of one part of the ego annihilating other parts which, I suggest, underlies the world catastrophe phantasy … implies a preponderance of the destructive impulse over the libido … If the ego and the internalized objects are felt by the infant to be in bits, an internal catastrophe is experienced which both extends to the external world and is projected on to it. Such anxiety states relating to internal catastrophe arise, … during the period of the infantile paranoid (or schizoid) position and form the basis for later schizophrenia. In Freud's view the dispositional fixation to Dementia Præcox is found in a very early stage of development. Referring to Dementia Præcox, which Freud distinguished from Paranoia, he said: 'The dispositional point of fixation must therefore be situated further back than in paranoia, and must

> lie somewhere at the beginning of the course of development from auto-erotism to object-love' (Freud, 1911, p. 464) … I suggest that the raid which ended in the Flechsig souls being reduced to one or two, was part of the attempt towards recovery. For the raid was to undo, one may say heal, the split in the ego by annihilating the split-off parts of the ego. As a result, only one or two of the souls were left which, as we may assume, were meant to regain their intelligence and their power. This attempt towards recovery, however, was effected by very destructive means used by the ego against itself and its introjected objects.
>
> *(Klein, 1946, pp. 109–110, emphasis in original)*

Fairbairn's paper on the Schreber case (1956) includes the following:

> the researches of Melanie Klein led her to the conclusion that the development of the super ego is effected through the integration … of a multiplicity of internalised part-objects, many of which are 'bad objects' and function as internal persecutors (Klein 1948). In accordance with this view, it becomes possible to understand how, in circumstances favouring regression, the superego may disintegrate into the internalised part-objects from which it originated, with the consequent release of a host of internal persecutors, and how such internal persecutors may be defensively projected into the external world (Klein 1948).
>
> *(Fairbairn, 1994[1956], p. 50)*

And later:

> Melanie Klein's conception of internal persecutors has, however, enabled the gap left in Freud's explanation of paranoia, to be filled; for, as she has pointed out: … the pains and other manifestations which in phantasy result from the attacks of the persecuting objects within against the ego are typically paranoid (Klein, 1948, pp. 292–293).
>
> *(Fairbairn, 1994[1956], p. 55)*

Red (Adelaide) returns / projects the internal persecutors to the external world and then sets about destroying the 'above grounders' in order to recover and restore her original state.

Freud concludes his paper on Schreber in the following way:

> This short postscript to my analysis of a paranoid patient may serve to show that Jung had excellent grounds for his assertion that the mythopoeic forces of mankind are not extinct, but that to this very day they give rise in the neuroses to the same psychical products as in the remotest past ages. I should like to take up a suggestion that I myself made some time ago and add that the same holds good of the forces that construct

> religions. And I am of opinion that the time will soon be ripe for us to make an extension of a thesis which has long been asserted by psycho-analysts, and to complete what has hitherto had only an individual and ontogenetic application by the addition of its anthropological counter-part, which is to be conceived phylogenetically. 'In dreams and in neu-roses', so our thesis has run, 'we come once more upon the child and the peculiarities which characterize his modes of thought and his emotional life.' 'And we come upon the savage too,' we may now add, 'upon the primitive man, as he stands revealed to us in the light of the researches of archaeology and of ethnology.'
>
> *(Freud, 1911, p. 82)*

All of which suggests to me that Red and Adelaide are both working from a deeply paranoid position. For Fairbairn, the transitional paranoid state is when the *Ideal Self* is kept internally but is threatened by attacks from the *Libidinal* and *Antilibidinal Selves* that are projected externally (Fairbairn, 1952, p. 46).

External Worlds

The humanist horror of Jordan Peele's American Nightmare

> … Obama came out of nowhere, nowhere. People who went to school with him, they never knew where he was from.
>
> *(Donald Trump on Obama's birth certificate)*

In a series of critical interviews and throughout much of his work, Jacques Derrida (1972) sets out how Western thought is predicated on binaries. Fol-lowing on from Saussure, he states that meaning is often defined in terms of binary oppositions, where "one of the two terms governs the other" (Derrida, 1972). In Trump's America, the binary fissures of race – the stark conflicts of black and white, which have defined the history of the union, have been vio-lently reopened throughout the entire summer of 2020 and into and beyond the disputed November election.

Race has driven Trump for more than 40 years. From the Justice Depart-ment racial discrimination case against his property company in 1973, to the 1989 full-page newspaper ads taken out by Trump arguing that the Central Park Five should be executed (strangely referenced in *Joker*) Trump's record on race is questionable, to say the least. The origin story of his unlikely but successful run to the White House was his very public and constant 'birth-erism' challenge of the Obama birth certificate. Trump certainly didn't start the 'birther' movement, which asserted that Obama wasn't born in America, but he gave it the highest-profile backing (Graham et al., 2019). It was one of the first blatant political lies that he successfully and repeatedly doubled down on – a foreshadowing of his style to come. As Kakutani (2018) says, Trump is "a candidate who launched his political career on the original sin of birtherism". Birth rights and the imposter are of course central to the twists in *Us.*

The 2020 US election was played out on a knife edge, as the 'them's' and 'us's' took up such distinctly different positions and versions of the truth. One thing is clear – the Trump / Biden election was as much about race as anything. As Snyder (2021) put it:

> it's not just that electoral fraud by African Americans against Donald Trump never happened. It is that it is the very opposite of what happened, in 2020 and in every American election. As always, Black people waited longer than others to vote and were more likely to have their votes challenged. They were more likely to be suffering or dying from Covid-19, and less likely to be able to take time away from work.

One common and simple way to put this opposition (following on from Edward Said (1993) and Derrida), is the concept of 'Them' and 'Us'. There is both 'us' (the opposite of them) and there is 'the US' (the United States), as Peele spells out when the two doppelganger families collide near the beginning of his film.

Us is the creation of Jordan Peele, a comedian, fan boy and writer / director, deeply steeped in popular culture, horror and sci-fi. Therefore, it won't have escaped Peele that *Them!* (1954) is a Cold War sci-fi film about nuclear ants that threaten to take over LA. They come home to roost ten years after being mutated in some bunkers in the desert, where the American military have been testing nuclear weapons.

Us starts with a similar idea – the legend at the opening spells out an underground experiment from Reagan's 1980s gone wrong. *Us* seems to be making a clear and metaphorical link from Reagan's America and the paranoid 1950s world of *Them* through to Trump's reimagined nostalgia for an America that never really existed, and which is symbolised by the ubiquitous MAGA hat.

Whilst *Them* spoke of the spectre of Communism, the Cold War and the threat of nuclear annihilation, *Us* is much more firmly linked to the horrors within ourselves and the underbelly of the American Dream itself. Like *Sicario*, it deals with borders, and much like Trump's insular foreign policy, it deals with the enemy on the border within – an internal enemy, figured externally in the film – the other (family).

Us is a film about doubles and doppelgangers – most particularly an African American family and their violent, vengeful other halves. It's also about the United States we know above ground and the United States we fear, that lurks below, the America of mass homelessness and poverty – for the middle class, its collective unconscious. This is an America that exists in the segregated and no-go areas of the big cities we never cross the tracks to – cities like Atlanta, Chicago and LA.

Us is Jordan Peele's second film as writer / director – a twisting rollercoaster of a film that dazzles en route with its audacity and ambition. Peele chooses the genre of horror, to reveal some large part of the American Dream's flipside – the American Nightmare. The absolute nightmare of race and class. The American Dream is that we are all born equal, imbued with some sense and mythology that 'we can do anything', but ultimately our socio-economic circumstances are more likely to leave us out in the cold.

Who is Jordan Peele?

Prior to 2016, Jordan Peele was primarily known as a comedian / writer, appearing regularly on his own sketch show, *Key and Peele*, but little had prepared anyone for the transformation that followed.

Peele burst into film in 2017, writing and directing *Get Out*, a horror thriller with an elevated twist on racism, and a powerful subtext about white liberal privilege and the Black Lives Matter movement itself. Within the story, the finger was pointed not at the easy and obvious target of Trump-supporting white Republicans but more significantly and less obviously at the privileged white liberals themselves. In *Get Out*, these are liberals who both eulogise the black body / form and steal it at the same time for their own purposes – a metaphor for the use and reification of black culture by white America if ever there was one. This was put to the sword by Wesley Morris in his article "For centuries, black music, forged in bondage, has been the sound of complete artistic freedom. No wonder everybody is always stealing it" (Morris, 2019).

By 2020, Peele had become one of the most powerful producers and directors in Hollywood. As significant as his race was that his Oscar was for a film in the horror genre, for a screenplay in the original category. *The Exorcist* was the only other horror screenplay to win as adapted screenplay, in 1973. *Get Out* therefore joined a small and brilliant oeuvre of original horror films that transcended the genre through social commentary and razor-tight execution (in America, a list that includes Kubrick's *The Shining*, Polanski's *Rosemary's Baby,* Friedkin's *The Exorcist*, De Palma's *Carrie* and Carpenter's *They Live.*)

Baldwin and the American Dream

Midway through the first episode of the Jordan Peele-produced *Lovecraft Country* (2020), the story is disrupted by the unexplained and unannounced non-diegetic sound of James Baldwin's address to the Cambridge University Union in 1965. It's one of the strangest moments I've seen on American television. The Baldwin address happened some ten years after the *Lovecraft County* narrative in question and is unexplained in the sense that we never see Baldwin, nor are we told who is speaking, or from where. It is a meta-commentary very much in line with Peele's work.

This is what we hear, and Baldwin said, in 1965:

> It would seem to me the proposition before the House, and I would put it that way, is the American Dream at the expense of the American Negro, or the American Dream is at the expense of the American Negro, is a question hideously loaded, and then one's response to that question – one's reaction to that question – has to depend on effect and, in effect, where you find yourself in the world, what your sense of reality is, what your system of reality is. That is, it depends on assumptions which we hold so deeply as to be scarcely aware of them.
>
> *(Baldwin, 1965)*

This is heard over the backdrop of the main character, Atticus, traveling across the 1950s Midwest – the crossing point between two halves of the American Dream itself, a fissure in the fabric of America that still exists today. (Despite the remarkable Stacey Abrams inspired results in Georgia, 2021 (Omara, A., 2020)). In fact, in the light of the Trump presidency and the Black Lives Matter movement, a fissure that was barely concealed during the Obama presidency (lest we forget Michael Brown and the Ferguson unrest of 2014 (*New York Times*, 2014)), and which has been ripped asunder by the events of the last few years, most prominently with the 2020 murder of George Floyd at the hands of the Minneapolis police.

In that 1965 Cambridge debate, between right-wing author and publisher William Buckley and James Baldwin, it was Baldwin who came out on top, not only by winning the vote, but morally as well. As he put it to the assembled students, "I picked the cotton, and I carried it to the market, and I built the railroads under someone else's whip for nothing. For nothing." (Baldwin, 1965).

It is Baldwin's examination of the American Dream that sits as importantly alongside Chomsky's (Chomsky, 2017). Baldwin was explicit about race and how much of the winners from the 'Dream' had benefited from endemic racial injustice. What, one might call, an internal colonialism in a country of immigrants that still exists to this day.

Written in 1835 and 1840, de Tocqueville's *Democracy in America* is a classic text containing commentary on both the Native Americans ("Indians" in de Tocqueville's work) and black people. We have already commented on the way that he sees the Native Americans while discussing the *Revenant.* What he writes about seems eerily prescient, and in keeping with much of Baldwin's work.

> The Indians will die in isolation as they have lived; but the destiny of the Negroes is in a way intertwined with that of the Europeans … The most dreadful of all the evils that threaten the future of the United States arises

> from the presence of blacks on its soil. When one seeks the cause of the present troubles and future dangers of the Union, from whatever point one departs one almost always arrives at this first fact … among the moderns the immaterial and fugitive fact of slavery is combined in the most fatal manner with the material and permanent fact of difference in race. The remembrance of slavery dishonors the race, and race perpetuates the remembrance of slavery … There is no African who has come freely to the shores of the New World, from which it follows that all those found there in our day are slaves or freedmen. Thus, the Negro transmits to all his descendants, with their existence, the external sign of his ignominy … The moderns, after having abolished slavery, therefore have still to destroy three prejudices much more intangible and more tenacious than it: the prejudice of the master, the prejudice of race, and finally the prejudice of the white … Those who hope that the Europeans will one day intermingle with Negroes therefore appear to me to cherish a chimera … Until now, everywhere that whites have been most powerful, they have held Negroes in degradation or in slavery. Everywhere that Negroes have been strongest, they have destroyed whites; this is the only account that has ever been opened between the two races … Racial prejudice appears to me stronger in the states that have abolished slavery than in those where slavery still exists, and nowhere is it shown to be as intolerant as in states where servitude has always been unknown … In almost all the states where slavery was abolished, the Negro has been given electoral rights; but if he presents himself to vote, he runs a risk to his life. Oppressed, he can complain, but he finds only whites among his judges… Thus, the Negro is free, but he can share neither the rights, nor the pleasures, nor the labors, nor the grief, nor even the tomb of the one whose equal he has been declared; nowhere can he meet with him, neither in life nor in death.
>
> *(De Tocqueville, Part 2 Section 10)*

It is this racial injustice allied with a humanism that sits at the heart of the Jordan Peele universe. From his interviews, this is a hermetically sealed universe that he has deliberately invented and created. It is markedly different to the universes of Marvel or DC or Star Wars, in that it is overtly, deliberately and allegorically political. It is trying to speak through Peele's love of the genre to racism and the horrors of American society.

The Baldwin speech is one of the few, if not the only, explicit expressions of what is at the heart of Peele's work. And that heart for Peele, I would argue, is the very nature of America's reality, the oppression of the African American (and the underclass) and the mythologies of the American Dream. Peele brilliantly uses the horror genre to speak about this racist America.

In 2020, Peele masterminded two shows, both with explicit roots and references in the 1950s. A reboot of the Rod Sterling 1959 anthology *The*

Twilight Zone for CBS and a strange take on 1950s America in the aforementioned HBO hit *Lovecraft Country* (based on the 2016 book). In popular culture, post-war 1950s America is often portrayed as an idyllic suburbia – the 'place of return' for Trump's MAGA-wearing zealots, but this decade was, uncoincidentally, also the starting point, through the actions of Rosa Parks, Malcolm X and Martin Luther King, for the nascent civil rights movement and the emergence of a young James Baldwin himself with his 1955 essay collection, *Notes of a Native Son*. Trump's exhortations seem a barely disguised call for a return to a world before the civil rights movement and its victories that ultimately saw Obama elected as president.

Like Baldwin, Peele wants to use his art to reveal what lies just under the surface of American society. As Johnny Pitts says of Baldwin in his book *Afropean* (2020),

> Baldwin was perhaps the most coherent literary voice of the civil rights struggle because he managed to present black people as humans … rather than mere actors in a polemic to hammer home a moralistic or political message. He made America see there was no hope of an American Dream unless it included everybody.

As Baldwin (2017) himself said, "You never had to look at me. I had to look at you. I know more about you than you know about me. Not everything that is faced can be changed, but nothing can be changed until it is faced."

Not far below the surface

In Peele's work it is the unmasking of reality – the revelation of what lies under the surface or beneath that is central to the story universe. The Peele mythologies of the 'Sunken Place' and the 'Underground' deal most explicitly with this. The suggestion is that something powerful lies beneath the veneer of the idea of America – and it is ready to break out.

America had been here before – most particularly, Los Angeles in 1992, but when, some 15 months after the release of *Us*, BLM riots broke out across the US, the film took on an even greater meaning. Trump's rhetoric, videos of police brutality and murder, the MAGA hats, the Proud Boys, the pent-up racism fuelled by the clickbait mania of surveillance capitalism, had driven America to the brink.

The Black Lives Matter movement became the ideological and actual battle ground not only for the 2020 election, but at times it seemed, the very soul of America. BLM had been an important but ultimately ineffectual side bar to the 2016 election, borne out of incidents of police brutality, specifically in Ferguson and Baltimore. The original flash point had been the death of Trayvon Martin in 2012, his murderer Zimmerman's acquittal in 2014, and the auction of the murder weapon by Zimmerman for $250,000 in 2016 – all adding fuel to the growing fire.

Following George Floyd's murder at the height of lockdown on 25 May 2020, and the video of his brutal arrest, protests spread across America and much of Europe too. There were large-scale gatherings, some violent, many peaceful, mid-Covid pandemic, from Portland to Paris.

Whilst Trump has undoubtedly increasingly fanned the flames this time, it is a fire that had begun to burn under the Obama administration, and like many of America's problems of race and class, not something that Trump alone created. As Baldwin and De Tocqueville remind us, it is a fire that has always burnt from the birth of the nation through to the present day.

It is a mistake, that the left continually return to, that without Trump, America would somehow be a racially and socially just country – but this is simply not the case.

Not enough has really changed since Baldwin's 1965 address – race, class and patriarchy remain at the heart of a now rising inequality across America.

Parasite, Shoplifters and Us

Peele followed the racially charged *Get Out*, with *Us*, a film that has much in common with Korea's Oscar winner, *Parasite* (Bong Joon-Ho, 2019) or Cannes Palme D'Or-winning film *Shoplifters* (Koreeda, 2018).

These three films take a look at class (and more precisely the disenfranchised underclass) with a withering and damning eye. All three shine a strange light on those left behind in the wake of neoliberalism – the 'dispossessed' become the main protagonists. All share much in common with the works of Dickens, or Twain's *Prince and the Pauper*. This coincidental thread of those 'who live below', that unites all three films, suggests that the problems of the underclass, at least, go beyond America.

Parasite, like *Us*, deals with the figurative / metaphorical problem of what monsters lurk below, and uses the doubling (and to some degree tripling) of families as a parable for the schism between those who have and have not. Whilst *Parasite* takes a masterful Hitchcockian thriller approach, and *Shoplifters* a heightened realist one, Peele's *Us* takes a more fantastical, complex genre approach.

There are significant links between the three films. In *Shoplifters* and *Parasite*, we get a picture of two tense Asian families who are united in their poverty and their need for ingenuity to survive. They live in cramped subterranean spaces. In the case of *Parasite*, the family lives precariously below the water line, where the toilets flood and other people's wi-fi can be stolen. In *Shoplifters*, the 'reveal' that these people are not related but together by necessity for survival makes us question what even makes a family. In *Parasite* and *Us* the audience is asked: how does the underclass family survive? Guile in both cases seems to be the answer – there is a sense of Darwinism run amok in these universes. Survival of the fittest – or the wiliest. Kill or be killed.

In *Us*, the link to this question of what makes a family is clear, whilst the two families in *Parasite* are mirrored metaphorically – rich and poor. In *Us* it is a literal as well as metaphorical doubling. Stairs underground to unknown undiscovered places unite these two films. the stairs / escalators we see in *Us* that lead to the underworld are doubled in the *Parasite* house, with its secret area downstairs (a shot-for-shot comparison of the stairs in both films is striking in their similarity, though neither was aware of the other in production).

> Stairs – and more specifically an escalator in *Us* – and basements show the audience the descent the characters take physically and mentally. In *Us*, young Adelaide plunges into the funhouse's dark recesses and deeper still in the forgotten underground train system where the tethered live. In *Parasite* it's the stairs connecting the posh, obscenely expensive furnished and decorated, living quarters of the Parks to the cold bunker Geun Se inhabits. Additionally, a series of external stairs in the Kim's neighborhood, demonstrate how far they actually live from their hope of wealth. It's down these flights of stairs that their dreams begin to wash away in a deluge of dirty, flooding rainwater.
>
> *(Hinds, C., 2020)*

Whilst *Parasite* was showered with praise and Oscars (unheard of for a foreign language film), *Us* was bizarrely overlooked, but undoubtedly featured one of the great performances of the decade by Lupita Nyong'o (as acknowledged by Richard Brody (2021)). The two films clearly speak to the same underlying anxiety – the problem of the underclass – those beneath the stairs. Is there a case to be made for the fact that Hollywood and the Academy struggled with *Us* and its virtuoso performance from Lupita Nyong'o, because it went to the heart of the class problem in America? The class problems of poverty, education, health and housing that exist in the 'refugee camp' – Skid Row – on the streets of Downtown LA and beyond. The prevalence of this problem, all over LA, seem to suggest that Hollywood may be unable to meaningfully confront these problems in its own back yard. Was *Parasite*, at one remove, easier to stomach than Peele's take on American race and class? Is the horror of the genre and the close-to-home horror of *Us* too uncomfortable? Are the saccharine race relations seen in *Crash* or *Green Book* far more palatable for the Academy and the Foreign Press Association? An idealised but unrealistic world where racist cops or security are transformed completely through relations with their black co-stars.

The horror of capitalism

Regardless of awards, *Us* makes a meaningful allegorical contribution to the argument that this is not just a Trumpian problem. It is clearly one that stretches at least as far back to the neoliberal roots of Reagan's America. Peele makes the time of the fissure in American society very specific through the prologue and its overt references to the aforementioned Reaganite charity show Hands Across America and Michael Jackson's Thriller – the 1980s. *Joker* also references this time in its own mish mash Gotham / NYC universe. Both films obliquely seem to suggest that the problem began in the Reagan years – the beginning of neoliberalism. Peele makes this explicit by stating that the origin of the problem was "government experiments from that period", clearly linking the tethered to the Reagan-inspired Hands Across America.

He also makes it clear that the people above ground embody the American Dream. The following exchange between Adelaide and Zora reflects these underlying belief systems of self-actualisation and meritocracy. Zora says that she is going to make it to the Olympics, and Adelaide agrees, saying that she can do anything she sets her mind to. But, Adelaide is shown to be wrong; Trump's chaotic presidency has taken the failed American Dream and accelerated its flipside. As Phipps says:

> Years from now, Peele's film will look like a document of how we lived during the Trump years, how each moment felt freighted with anxiety about what will come next and whether or not we'll survive it. It's a film about now, and about us.
>
> *(Phipps, 2020)*

Peele understands the American Dream is built on an American Nightmare: that there are a those 'who have', and a growing number in America who have not. Racism has always been an essential facet of achieving the dream. America, as Baldwin and De Tocqueville saw, was built on the backs of the non-whites, the underclass and the working class. In *Us*, as well as the racial divide, the class war is symbolised by the tethered and their wealthy doppelgangers above ground. It is a reminder that affluence, like race, is an accident of birth and that American capitalism, particularly neoliberalism stretching back to Reagan, isn't working. Many are excluded. In *Us*, the tethered are a reflection of who we might be, who we might become if we lost our jobs, or became sick, or suffered racism. Those left behind in an increasingly divided world of them and us.

References

Bailey, J. (2019) 'The Story of Hands Across America, the Failed Fundraiser Featured in Jordan Peele's *Us*'. *Vulture*. https://www.vulture.com/2019/03/hands-across-america-in-jordan-peele-s-us.html

Baldwin , *J.* (1965) 'Baldwin debates Buckley'. *YouTube*. https://www.youtube.com/watch?v=oFeoS41xe7w

Baldwin, J. (2017) *I Am Not Your Negro*. London: Penguin.

Brody, R. (2021) 'The Best Movie Performances of the Century so far'. *The New Yorker*.

Chomsky, N. (2017) *Requiem for the American Dream: The 10 Principles of Concentration of Wealth & Power*. Seven Stories Press.

Derrida, J. (1972 rep 2004) *Positions.* London: Continuum.
Fairbairn, W. R. D. (1952) *Psychoanalytic Studies of the Personality.* London: RKP.
Fairbairn, W. R. D. (1994) 'The Schreber Case'. In *From Instinct to Self*, eds. Scharff and Birtles (Vol I). Originally published as, 'Considerations Arising out of the Schreber Case'. The British Journal of Medical Psychology (1956), 29 (2): 113–127.
Freud, S. (1911) *Psycho-Analytic Notes on an Autobiographical Account of a Case of Paranoia (Dementia Paranoides). S.E. XII (1911–1913): The Case of Schreber, Papers on Technique and Other Works*, 1–82.
Graham, D. et al. (2019) *'An Oral History of Trump's Bigotry', The Atlantic.*
Hands across America (2015) https://web.archive.org/web/20150713191701/http://www.usaforafrica.org/Hands_Across_America/index.html.
Hinds, C. (2020) 'How Parasite and Us Both Reveal the Darkness of Social Inequality'. *The Observer.* https://observer.com/2020/04/us-parasite-bong-joon-ho-jordan-peele/.
House, W. (2017) 'We Can't Ignore H.P. Lovecraft's White Supremacy – Lovecraftian Narratives of Race Persist in Contemporary Politics'. *Lithub.*
Jones, E. E. (2020) 'Inside Cinema, 1: Jordan Peele'. *BBC.*
Jones, K. (2020) 'How Can We Win?'. *Youtube.* https://youtu.be/ZkedkvNn5V0
Kakutani, M. (2018) *The Death of Truth.* William Collins
Klein, M. (1946) 'Notes on Some Schizoid Mechanisms'. *International Journal of Psycho-Analysis*, 27: 99–110.
Klein, M. (1948) *Contributions to Psycho-analysis.* London: Hogarth.
Morris, W. (2019) 'For centuries, black music, forged in bondage, has been the sound of complete artistic freedom. No wonder everybody is always stealing it'. *The New York Times*, August.
National Geographic (n.d.) 'The Underground Railroad'. https://www.nationalgeographic.org/encyclopedia/underground-railroad/
New York Times (1987) 'Hands across America: Reach exceeded Grasp'. https://www.nytimes.com/1987/05/26/us/hands-across-america-rach-exceeded-grasp.html
New York Times Staff (2014) 'What happened in Ferguson?' *The New York Times*, August. https://www.nytimes.com/interactive/2014/08/13/us/ferguson-missouri-town-under-siege-after-police-shooting.html.
Omara, A. (2020) 'Democrats have Stacey Abrams to thank'. *The Independent*, November.
Phipps, K. (2020) 'Jordan Peele's Us, and the Other Films That Captured the Trump Era'. *GQ Magazine.* https://www.gq.com/story/trump-era-movies-us-borat-parasite-the-hunt#intcid=_gq-bottom-recirc_489b3814-90a0-401e-87d5-6bf28de3ae91_text2vec1.
Pitts, J. (2020) *Afropean.* London: Penguin.
Said, E. (1994) *Culture and Imperialism.* Vintage.
Snyder, T. (2021) 'The American Abyss'. *The New York Times*, January. https://www.nytimes.com/2021/01/09/magazine/trump-coup.html
Tocqueville de, A. (2000) *Democracy in America.* Translated, edited and with an introduction by H. C. Mansfield and D. Winthrop. University of Chicago Press.
Wells, H. G. (2005) *The Time Machine (Penguin Classics).* London: Penguin Books.

11

ONCE UPON A TIME IN HOLLYWOOD (TARANTINO, 2019)

The Way I See Things

Internal Worlds

Introduction

Once Upon a Time in Hollywood is a complex film. It is Quentin Tarantino's, ninth, maybe last, movie. 'The 9th film from Quentin Tarantino features a large ensemble cast and multiple storylines in a tribute to the final moments of Hollywood's golden age' (IMDB). The film is a counterfactual, alternative reality that shares much with the explicit setting and date of the original action but has passed through the looking glass to become a 'wish fulfilling' alternative history. Remembering Fairbairn's comments that "dreams are essentially, not wish-fulfilments, but snapshots, or rather 'shorts' (in the cinematographic sense), of situations existing in inner reality", we might argue that this alternative history functions to preserve Sharon Tate as a *Libidinal Self* and that the internal dynamic between putative *Central Selves* comes down on the side of Rick as the preferred choice rather than Cliff.

Reading the film using Fairbairn's theory of dreams as representing elements of endopsychic structure leads us fairly quickly to the idea that, at the heart of the film / dream, there is a double figure who might be considered as a candidate for the *Central Self* – Rick Dalton, ageing TV and movie star, and his sidekick and stunt-double, Cliff Booth.

If these are to be considered as potential *Central Selves*, then the end of the film might indicate which of the two was the real *Central Self* and which a failed, or defunct *Central Self*. At the end, Rick is about to visit next-door neighbour, Sharon Tate, wife of Roman Polanski, with Jay Sebring. Rick and Cliff have just survived a murderous attack on Rick's house by three hippies from the Manson gang, thanks, in the main, to the courage and bravery of

DOI: 10.4324/9781003206224-12

Cliff and his pitbull, Brandy. Cliff has been taken off to hospital in an ambulance, and the last thing that Rick says to him is that he is a good friend, to which Cliff responds with a shrug, saying that he tries.

At the beginning of the film, Rick and Cliff see Polanski and Tate in their MG sports car entering the next-door drive. Rick waxes lyrical about Polanski as the director of *Rosemary's Baby* and fantasises about going to a pool party with them and securing a part in one of Polanski's movies. The end, in this alternative reality, would seem to suggest that Rick may be about to achieve this dream, a part in a Polanski movie that would be a fillip for his career. A career which he has resuscitated by going to make films as a leading man in Italy, as suggested by an agent (Al Pacino); the move from TV westerns in the 1950s to spaghetti westerns in the 1960s being a well-trodden and successful path, for some at least. It turns out that when he returns, Rick has married an Italian film star, so he has moved closer to the type of showbiz couple that his response to Polanski and Tate suggested is his ideal.

His newfound status and expensive lifestyle, coupled with the diminishing amount of work he can find for Cliff means that this last night is the parting of their ways. Even if he does go and visit Cliff in hospital next day and "bring bagels", as Cliff suggests, the days of their close working together, of Cliff giving up any ambitions he may have had in order to help and support Rick, are over. On the principle of 'last man standing' the *Central Self* is Rick, and Cliff is out of the picture.

This matters because they are very different models for a *Central Self*, and the loss of Cliff as part of a schizoid *Central Self* is a significant loss. In Winnicottian terms, it is as if the false self took over and the true self was lost.

Other reviewers of this film have also identified significant differences between the two putative *Central Selves*. We will use Roger Ebert's website as typical of the distinctions they make. Rick is: "keenly aware that his days of heroism are ending as he ages out of Hollywood … Cliff is way more laid-back, the kind of guy who loves his dog almost as much as he loves Rick and says what he means even to someone like Bruce Lee" (Tallerico, 2019).

Comment

The critics', opinions drawn from a small number of reviews, seem to all be of a similar viewpoint that, of the two, Rick is the most vulnerable, needy and insecure, while Cliff is the more mature, competent, and realistic and the one in this relationship who is doing all the giving. Cliff has no interest in a career and devotes his time to helping Rick in whatever ways he can. Rick, lacking self-confidence, is surely less mature, more infantile, while Cliff, who is supremely self-confident, is maturely dependent and capable of behaving in an adult fashion towards others.

Two examples of this are when Cliff has picked up the hitchhiking underage 'Pussycat' and she offers to fellate him while they are driving to the Spahn ranch. She is shocked that Cliff asks her for ID to prove that she is of legal age and taunts him with the suggestion that he is impotent, to which he replies that he has managed to stay out of jail so far and he is not going to risk it for 'poontang'. He may be doing this to prevent himself from being arrested and charged with the rape of a minor, so, acting in his own self-interest, but when he insists upon seeing George, who owns the Spahn ranch, because he thinks that the hippies living there may be forcing him to let them stay there and using his property against his will, this is Cliff looking out for a former friend and incurring danger in the process. A lesser man might have walked away without braving the hippies' antagonism, after having been consensually fellated by an underage girl.

There is little or no indication in the final scenes that anything has changed within either Rick or Cliff, so, if these two part, on a more or less permanent basis, the *Central Self* will have been weakened and hollowed out; will be less mature and capable than before. Rick is likely to continue as before in the film business, without the support of Cliff but with the support of his film star wife, whereas Cliff, who can look after himself, will find some way that he can flourish, some other good cause to put his energies into. This raises the question of the *Ideal Selves* of these two possible *Central Selves.*

Ideal Selves

For Rick his *Ideal Self*, or perhaps 'idealised' self would be a better description, would be to live like Polanski and Tate – a successful Hollywood marriage as they were at the time; a time that, through this alternative history, is preserved. A future chapter in that story might be of a film that Polanski makes starring Rick Dalton and Sharon Tate. That, at any rate, is the tenor of Rick's imagination and aspirations, success in the film business at a high level.

Cliff, on the other hand, has more demanding ideals; ideals he imposes on his dog, who is trained to overcome its impulses and wait for his appropriate command. So too with his willing ability to do what is required for Rick without resentment, alongside his refusal to be talked down to, or to defer, if he doesn't feel that it is warranted. His ability to fight his own corner, stand by his own principles, be his own man, all of which have led to his bad reputation and his difficulty getting work.

With Cliff's disappearance, the values to be admired and valued become the empty values of the commercial Hollywood world, celebrity and stardom, money and fame. It is perhaps significant that the black and white TV excerpts from *Bounty Law* depicting 'Jake Cahill', Rick's most memorable character, remembered warmly by everyone from Polanski and Tate to the hippies, is a ruthless killer for his own profit. The last shots of Rick are of his playing Jake Cahill advertising Red Apple cigarettes, cigarettes he patently hates and spits out, after delivering the advertising slogan for the no doubt fat cheque. Unprincipled to the end and perhaps an echo of the Marlboro man's destiny to come.

The *Libidinal* and *Antilibidinal Selves (Internal Saboteur)*: The Over-Exciting and Over-Rejecting Selves

The easiest personifications to identify, in that Rick gives us our lead on a number of occasions, mouthing off at the "fucking hippy scum" standing on a street corner, are the hippies as an over-exciting (libidinal) and an over-rejecting (aggressive) group threatening the status quo for Rick and for mainstream America. Rick's resentful outburst follows the speculations by his putative agent Schwarz (Pacino), that the networks might have been manipulating Rick's career for their own ends, which has nudged Rick to the conclusion that his career is over, leading to tears in the car park, which Cliff covers with his dark glasses and the admonition not to let the Mexican car park attendants see him crying.

This is followed by a dramatic reversal of Rick's mood, as he and Cliff pull up to Rick's house and see next-door neighbours Polanski and Tate driving into their house, Rick imagining that he might make it into one of Polanski's films one day by attending a pool party at his neighbours.

We witness the hippy's antilibidinal behaviour at the Spahn ranch and outside Rick's house before we witness what might be the hysterical displacement of Tarantino's anger at the hippies for killing Sharon Tate. This black comedic revenge on the hippies is difficult to make sense of but speaks of a tremendous resentment at the death of Sharon Tate and her friends and the effect that it, and the wider hippie movement, had on American sensibilities.

As for the libidinal aspects, the over-exciting spectacle of young, barely clad girls offering sex without strings was clearly a part of both the 1960s and the Manson family. That this sex was in no sense 'free love' but sex as manipulation and power is also part of the overlap between the libidinal and the antilibidinal, the over-exciting and the over-rejecting. It is thus also a part of what Marcuse called 'repressive desublimation' (Marcuse, [1964] 2002).

This uprising of exemplars of both libidinal and antilibidinal motivations and powers threatens the received wisdoms of both Rick and Cliff as *Central Selves*, so when one of the older women at the Spahn ranch says innocently of the girl Pussycat that they all love Pussy, Cliff can respond enthusiastically with a twinkle in his eye, despite having spurned the girl's advances earlier, on principled grounds.

Mature Dependence

It is clear from the first that Cliff is the one who is maturely dependent, whereas Rick remains sometimes painfully insecure, stuttering, tearful and unable to develop or achieve maturity. Without money or star status, Cliff is from the beginning his own man, not locked into self-serving machismo, but someone who can read situations accurately and respond realistically to them even if it exposes him to some risk. He is also free of the self-doubt and self-criticism that cripples Rick's ability to perform, and Rick's emotional fragility is knowingly highlighted by Tarantino when he has Rick glowing in response to the praise he receives for his acting from a precocious eight-year-old starlet, wise beyond her years. Rick's progress from fading TV star to rejuvenated leading man with a potential connection to Hollywood 'royalty' is no solution for his fractured self, while Cliff, injured, abandoned and with no firm job or future, is nevertheless confident of his ability to flourish in this world because he sees the world clearly and can act appropriately no matter what is thrown at him, literally or metaphorically.

The whispered story of Cliff killing his wife and getting away with it, is illustrated by the ambiguous scene leading up to the, perhaps accidental, shooting of his wife with a harpoon gun, while she is belittling and criticising him on board a small fishing boat. While Rick is constantly subject to 'ressentiment' in particular towards hippies, both individually and as a group, Cliff has no such feelings. Cliff is careful to check that his former friend at the Spahn ranch, who seems to be being exploited by the hippies, is all right, despite the dangers he has to face in insisting he see his friend, but once satisfied that he is OK he walks away, after making one of the hippies, who has stuck a knife in one of his tyres, change the wheel.

> Ressentiment is a vengeful, petty-minded state of being that does not so much want what others have (although that is partly it) as want others to not have what they have. The term, which might be translated as 'resentment', though in most places it is generally left in the original French, is usually associated with German philosopher Friedrich Nietzsche, who defined it as a slave morality. Nietzsche sees *ressentiment* as the core of Christian and Judaic thought and, consequently, the central facet of western thought more generally. In this context, *ressentiment* is more fully defined as the desire to live a pious existence and thereby position oneself to judge others, apportion blame, and determine responsibility. Nietzsche did not invent the concept of *ressentiment*, it was a term that was very much 'in the air' in his lifetime (the late 19th century), as Fredric Jameson points out in his sharp critique of the concept in *The Political Unconscious* (1981). Jameson's quarrel with *ressentiment*, or more particularly Nietzsche's deployment of it, is that the latter fails to consider the ideological weight the term carried in its own time; thus, in Jameson's view Nietzsche fails to see that it is a category deployed by the ruling bourgeoisie elite to simultaneously justify their privileges and rationalize the denial of those same privileges to the poorer classes (on

this view of things, the masses revolt not because their cause is just, but because they resent the rich).

(*Oxford Reference*)

This would seem to be the role that the hippies play for Rick, and by extension Tarantino, which might go some way to explaining the ending of the film. Rick doesn't want what the hippies have, which is a chimerical and chemical freedom, but he resents their apparent freedom to do what they want because he has had to work hard for whatever he has achieved, with the considerable but underacknowledged assistance of Cliff. Meanwhile, friendship with and a role in a possible film directed by Polanski and starring Sharon Tate, with leading man Rick, represents, for Rick, the final fantasy of acceptance into the Hollywood Hall of fame.

Conclusion

The old certainties of the post-war 1950s are being replaced by the chaos of unbridled emotions, libidinal and aggressive, that the hippies represented in different ways for both Rick and Cliff. The *Central Self* is being marginalised or eroded or becoming lost in the showbiz glitz and glamour of celebrity. The unconscious *Libidinal* and *Antilibidinal Selves* are erupting into the daylight and the ideals of an older generation are being dismantled.

Regarding this alternative narrative to the brutal murder of the heavily pregnant Sharon Tate and her friends, no magical attempt at rewriting history will succeed. The film stands in the same relationship to the reality as Karl Marx says of world history, at the opening of his article *The Eighteenth Brumaire of Louis Bonaparte* (1852), "Hegel remarks somewhere that all the events and personalities of great importance in world history occur, as it were, twice. He forgot to add the first time as tragedy, the second as farce."

This is a farcical (but masterful) retelling of a moment in history that in retrospect may be a tipping point for the American Dream, along with the murders of JFK, Malcolm X, Martin Luther King, and Bobby Kennedy, the landings on the moon. The whole film, in leading to a fantasy outcome, personified by Rick's story, is a pyrrhic victory.

External Worlds

A Tarantino film

As with the work of such iconic directors as Kubrick, Hitchcock or Leone, it's hard not to recognise a Tarantino film. However, two of my three favourite Tarantino films are not even purely his – Tony Scott's brilliant interpretation of his script *True Romance* and Tarantino's own empathetic and, unusually for him, emotional, adaptation of Elmore Leonard's *Jackie Brown*. He has remained, since the brilliant *Reservoir Dogs* (my other favourite) through to his self-declared ninth film *Once Upon a Time in Hollywood*, true to himself and his avowedly bombastic style. A style that redefined film-making cool in the 1990s, cherry-picking as it did from world and genre cinema, as the nerdy video-store cineaste Tarantino ruled Hollywood with his pop cultural offerings. Whilst the world and America got 9/11, the financial crash and the pandemic, Hollywood suffered the end of the DVD indie boom, the rise of the superhero blockbuster, the ascendancy of the streamers and then the much-needed Me Too and Time's Up movements that were provoked by the fall of Harvey Weinstein, producer of all but one of Tarantino's films. A number of other Hollywood figures, most notably Kevin Spacey, Armie Hammer and Woody Allen, were put under the spotlight and to some degree, in the parlance of the times, 'cancelled'. Relevant to *Once Upon a Time in Hollywood (OUATIH)*, as he is central to the plot, Roman Polanski, who had fled America to France the day before his sentencing in "an unlawful sex with a minor" case in 1977, was also put under the lens by the Me Too movement. This torrid story is well documented, most recently in the aforementioned examination of *Chinatown – The Big Goodbye* (Wassan, 2020).

It is hard to separate Quentin Tarantino, the man, from the film (*OUATIH*), set as it is in 1969 when he would have been six and living in Los Angeles with his single mother. The Manson-Tate murders took place in August of that year, up in Laurel Canyon, above the Sunset Strip. Tarantino is a director steeped in film culture and Hollywood history, having lived through much of it as an auteur over the last 30 years, and as a nerdy cineaste before that. Is it not strange, then, that at the height of the Me Too movement and controversy about his former producer Weinstein and the long-running Polanski extradition case, a man he once defended on the Howard Stern radio show, that he should write a film re-examining the murder of Polanski's pregnant wife Sharon Tate? *The Big Goodbye*'s (Wassan, 2020) opening line offers one possible surface reason – "Sharon Tate looked like California" and Tarantino just loves old California. Of course, historical revisionism is not new to Tarantino, as Jack Black points out,

> From 2009 to 2015, U.S. director, Quentin Tarantino released three films that were notable for their focus on particular historical events, periods and individuals (Inglorious Basterds 2009; Django Unchained 2012; The Hateful Eight 2015) Together these films offered a specifically 'Tarantinian' rendering of history – rewriting, manipulating and for some, unethically deploying history for aesthetic effect.
>
> *(Black, 2019, p. 1)*

The Manson murders are radically reimagined in *Once Upon a Time in Hollywood* such that the protagonists Cliff and Rick save Sharon Tate and her friends on that fateful August 1969 night on Cielo Drive. Tarantino's revisionist history was employed before in *Inglorious Basterds*, in which the plot to kill Hitler in a cinema came to a successful but unreal bloody fruition. Anything is possible in a post-truth world it seems, and life and cinema are for Tarantino completely intertwined. Oddly not featured in *Once Upon a Time in Hollywood* given the breadth of real characters in the film is Tate's friend Joan Didion. She knew Polanski well and interviewed one of the Tate killers Linda Kasabian in her definitive record of the time, *The White Album.* In her earlier work *Slouching Towards Bethlehem* (1968), Didion notes in her inimitable style, "This is the country in which a belief in the literal interpretation of Genesis has slipped imperceptibly into a belief in the literal interpretation of *Double Indemnity.*"

In *The White Album* (1979) she writes,

> Many people I know in Los Angeles believe that the Sixties ended abruptly on August 9, 1969, ended at the exact moment when word of the murders on Cielo Drive travelled like brushfire through the community, and in a sense this is true. The tension broke that day. The paranoia was fulfilled.

Tarantino and his ninth film are the bastard children of these two Didion quotes. Tarantino calls *Once Upon a Time in Hollywood* his "hang out" movie. In this, he seems to mean we get to spend a lot of time with Sharon Tate and the invented actor / stuntman buddies Rick and Cliff as they pass one particular day, earlier in 1969. Tate watches herself on screen, we see Rick acting, having a breakdown filming a TV western and then excusing his dangerous on-set behaviour with a minor, another strange choice for Tarantino given the recently resurfaced controversy around Uma Thurman's car crash on the set of *Kill Bill 2*. Later in the film, Cliff, while visiting the Manson ranch and checking in on the owner, congratulates himself on *not* having underage sex with one of the Manson hippy gang.

Once Upon a Time in Hollywood is a long film, some 2 hours and 40 minutes, with a four-hour version threatened for Netflix. But in the 40 minutes or so it took me to re-read Didion's *The White Album* I felt like I got much more a sense of the time, beyond its look, and while there's no doubt *OUATIH* is a stylishly directed postmodern film, it is also a bit like its stars Brad and Leo, great looking and full of swagger. Tarantino is undoubtedly a master filmmaker with huge resources at his fingertips, but this yarn meanders towards a brutal fantasist revisionist ending via hippy-bashing and reification of the white heterosexual machismo of Rick and Cliff. Made as it is at the height of the Me Too movement, it feels misjudged, Tarantino's timing out of joint.

The White Album of course references Manson's own obsession with the Beatles and particularly the track "Helter Skelter", which he saw as foreshadowing a coming race war between black and white. Manson's politics and hashed-up biblical, right-wing philosophy were not of the hippy movement, but like many since, the character of Josh Brolin's Matt in *Sicario* (Chapter 7) for instance, Manson co-opted their style because it suited his lust for power. Only three years before the murders, that elusive seer of white enclave Manhattan Beach, Thomas Pynchon had ventured east to Watts during the 1966 race riots. His article *A Journey into the Mind of Watts* echoes Didion's *Double Indemnity* assertion, contextualising the ignorance and prejudice around race in the city, revelatory for more than just his use of the word 'negro':

> For Los Angeles, more than any other city, belongs to the mass media. What is known around the nation as the L.A. Scene exists chiefly as images on a screen or TV tube, as four-color magazine photos, as old radio jokes, as new songs that survive only a matter of weeks. It is basically a white Scene, and illusion is everywhere in it, from the giant aerospace firms that flourish or retrench at the whims of Robert McNamara, to the 'action' everybody mills long the Strip on weekends looking for, unaware that they, and their search which will end, usually, unfulfilled, are the only action in town.
>
> Watts lies impacted in the heart of this white fantasy. It is, by contrast, a pocket of bitter reality. The only illusion Watts ever allowed itself was to believe for a long time in the white version of what a Negro was supposed to be. But with the Muslim and civil-rights movements that went, too.
>
> *(Pynchon, 1966)*

It should not surprise us, then, that Tarantino's ode to his idealised childhood and the way the movie business was, runs through just a narrow rectangle of LA from Topanga Canyon and Santa Monica to Hollywood via Beverly Hills and Laurel Canyon. An area of the city that was and remains largely white and segregated. Significantly, despite tensions in the city as bad as those of the recent BLM protests, Manson is vilified here, but not for being a harbinger of vicious racism, rather, as a "hippy". Contrast this with Pynchon's novel *Inherent Vice* (Pynchon, 2010) as adapted for the screen by fellow Angeleno P. T. Anderson (2014) – a book and film that stand in stark opposition to QT – and celebrates the hippy spirit of the era via its protagonist Doc Sportello (as played by Joaquin Phoenix). As Jen Chaney points out when examining Rick's pejorative use of the word and tirade against the long-haired of LA:

> What he is really mad at, of course, is time and the fact that it continues to move forward against his will, making him less and less relevant. But like most middle-aged or older folks who are really mad at time, he projects those feelings onto people who have more time than he does: the hippies, a.k.a. the young people rattling the status quo circa 1969 … Charles Manson and the brainwashed members of the Manson family technically were not hippies. They were killer sheep in hippie clothing. Actual hippies were not murderers. They were Vietnam War protesters and left-leaning peace advocates; pot smokers and acid droppers; free-

> love proponents who wore flowers in their hair and danced naked in the mud at Woodstock – which, for the record, took place a mere week after the Manson murders … They also were the rejecters of mainstream society who questioned the rules under which it operated.
>
> *(Chaney, 2019)*

On Franklin Avenue

Tarantino operates in an enclosed movie universe, a world that is self-referential, with each film he becomes more and more a mirror to himself – solipsistic to a degree and out of touch with the post-Weinstein world.

Here in *OUATIH*, Tarantino is at great pains and spares no expense creating the streets of Hollywood in period detail. In 1969, Didion lived on Franklin Avenue, right by Hollywood haunt, *El Coyote* (the last place Tate ate at before her murder) and the other restaurants and bars so lovingly recreated for the film. It is the same block of Franklin Avenue where Rita first finds herself, having been thrown from a mysterious car at the beginning of *Mulholland Drive.* But Didion and Lynch's Hollywood's jar with that of Tarantino. Lynch's doubling masterpiece speaks in a dream-like style of the corruption and misogyny of Hollywood in a way that *OUATIH* takes great pains to avoid. It is not Hollywood or its dreaming that's the problem for Tarantino, it's the world outside it. Tarantino seems to like it just the way it was, the way it used to be before those hippies and Me Too fanatics came to spoil the never-ending permanent vacation party of Hollywood.

Once Upon a Time...

Tarantino's *Once Upon a Time in Hollywood* of course also inevitably invokes Sergio Leone's two great 'Once Upon a Time' movies – *Once Upon a Time in the West (1968)* and *Once Upon a Time in America* (1984). Tarantino speaks of Leone glowingly in an essay for *The Spectator* (and an introduction to a book about Leone) when he describes how modern film students react to Leone's work:

> That's when they start recognising the elements. That's when they're not just 'I'm looking at an older movie now.' It's the use of music, the use of the set piece, the ironic sense of humour. They appreciate the surrealism, the craziness, and they appreciate the cutting to music. So, it is the true beginning of what filmmaking had evolved to by the 1990s. You don't go past Leone; you start with Leone.
>
> *(Tarantino, 2019)*

The influence on Tarantino of Leone's work is most keenly felt in his use of music. Leone was one of the first directors to ask his composer, Ennio Morricone to make the music and then film to it (as opposed to the other way around). Famously, he would choreograph shots to Morricone's operatic scores. When Stanley Kubrick asked Leone how the crane that introduces us to the fictional railroad town of Flagstone (in *Once Upon a Time in the West*) was timed so perfectly to the music, Leone explained that the score was already available on-set.

Alongside his inventive use of genre, his bravura pop cultural dialogue, his machismo characters and his revenge fantasies, it is Tarantino's use of music that he will be remembered for. The musical accompaniment of Stealers Wheel over the ear-slashing scene of *Reservoir Dogs*, the Chuck Berry dance in *Pulp Fiction* and *Jackie Brown*'s intro to Bobby Womack's 110th Street are all very much a part of the pop culture canon of the 90s. Later, as Tarantino became obsessed with his historical fictions and westerns (*Inglorious Basterds, Django Unchained, The Hateful Eight* and *OUATIH*) he even started to use old Morricone scores and then employed the master himself to compose his final score for *The Hateful Eight*. In the latter half of Tarantino's career, undoubtedly no director's presence is felt more keenly than Sergio Leone's.

Leone's *Once Upon a Time in the West* was released in 1968. It tells the story of the original American Dream, of the building of the railroad, of rape and murder and revenge, and of the old guard of ruthless men who fought to control the new Western Frontier. A kind of sequel to *The Revenant* of how brutally the West was won. *Once Upon a Time in America* begins and ends in the same year – 1968, looping back across the lives of four young Jewish kids in the lower East Side of New York from 1918 through to the prohibition and then up to the year of revolution 1968. A muzak version of the Beatles hit *Yesterday* bridges the gaps in time in the films epic time-hopping narrative. It is Leone's alternative to Coppola's *Godfather*, more European in its sublime, opium drenched use of time and space.

1968 was of course the year of revolution across the world. A revolution in America that saw the assassinations of Robert Kennedy (a few miles south of Hollywood Blvd) and Martin Luther King. Conversely, 1969 was the beginning of the end of that attempted revolution, and the immediate period that followed, post-Vietnam, Watergate and oil shock through to Reagan's election, saw the establishment of the neoliberal, postmodern and globalised era that we are still living through today. As Koraljka Suton puts it in the excellent *Beyond Cinephilia* (2019),

> In *Once Upon a Time in America*, Leone deals with the illusion of the American Dream, as seen through the eyes of Jewish kids whose entire childhoods are drenched in poverty, with the prospect of crime being the only logical solution, for which there exist no feelings of remorse or guilt. It is a visceral depiction of toxic masculinity which still reigns supreme in today's world, showing inherently broken children rising to power through violence and corruption. It is also a painfully accurate portrayal of inexcusable misogyny which was once considered a norm, with acts of violence (sexual and otherwise) against women shown in great detail and with little to no restraint. It is also a story of a man who feels inferior to

the woman he claims to love, leading him to exercise his dominance the only way he knows how – and resulting in her leaving him behind to make use of her talents and build a respectable life and career for herself.

By any standards, the sexual politics of both of Leone's films are retrograde and clearly sexist. Leone's slim get-out is the time he made these, a much harder case for Tarantino to make for his *Once Upon a Time*.... Leone's *Once Upon a Time*... films at least understand and explain the American Dream – the political corruption, the betrayals, the racism and the misogyny that underpin it. Like De Tocqueville, Baldwin, Dos Passos, Chomsky and Didion, Leone also shows the tragedy of the Dream that was broken before it was ever even realised.

Tarantino's sense of a dream is exactly that. Everything is on the surface. Nothing matters more than other movies. That the moment (1969) was important for Hollywood is hardly revelatory, but Tarantino's uncritical romanticising of the toxic masculinity of cowboy actors Rick and Cliff seems to be made (deliberately or inadvertently) for the tone deaf. Watts may as well be another country and Manson a plot device for the post-truth generation, or an excuse for more gratuitous vengeful violence.

It's difficult to reconcile this with Tarantino's own personal history and the present moment in cinema and America. *Once Upon a Time in Hollywood* is a movie that presents hanging out in the 1960s as "a gas", largely ruined by Manson and his hippy cohorts. If only it hadn't ended. Is this Tarantino's feeling writ large about the end of the indie days of Weinstein et al., the era before the streamers and Time's Up, or just his innocent playing around with history and a period he loved as a kid? It's impossible to say, but it feels like a film by a man out of time, as opposed to a film about what the end of the 1960s really meant. In the era of 'culture wars', Trump and his supporters' dangerous nostalgia for a 'make AMERICA great again' pre-civil rights era, it seems that Tarantino's narrative is careless at best.

Once Upon a Time in Hollywood ends with the brutal and graphic murder of the Manson gang, who in real life horribly murdered Tate and her friends. In this version, Rick and Cliff come to the rescue with flame throwers, and this grisly act of revenge or self-defence is the 'fairy tale' ending to the Tate story that Tarantino wants us to imagine. Like most of his films, revenge, the law of the talion, plays a big part in the drive of the story (most notably *Kill Bill* but also *Django Unchained, The Hateful Eight, Reservoir Dogs, Inglorious Basterds* and the 'Zed's dead' section of *Pulp Fiction*).

Revenge for 9/11, against Bin Laden and against a black president most notably, has driven American politics in the twenty-first century. Tarantino's films, as brilliantly crafted as they are, are sadly part of this pointless and endemic revenge culture and cycle. The violence is played for laughs and irony. As Postman said in *Amusing Ourselves to Death* (2006), "Orwell feared the truth would be concealed from us. Huxley feared it would be drowned in a sea of irrelevance." If endings are important to the meaning of a film, and tell us how seriously we should take them, what can we read back from Tarantino's ninth film?

> To go back to Andrew Sarris's policy, the stress on how can help us forget the what. Quentin Tarantino is not just a talented, film-mad kid. He is a citizen going from the twentieth to the twenty-first centuries and advocate for a woeful ideology. Film is not a closed room, a chamber for dreaming. It has to be part of the whole house of the nation.
>
> … In *Once Upon a Time*, the violence has to be held back for the big finish, a slap-up job. Anything else will be a cheat. The reviews didn't get into this because that would be a spoiler. Don't settle for that excuse. The film is so spoiled, it is beyond protection.
>
> *(Thompson, 2020, pp. 178, 182)*

Leone's final movie, *Once Upon a Time in America* ends somewhat differently. As Max says to Noodles (whom he has called back to kill, but Noodles refuses), "Is this your way of getting revenge?" De Niro's Noodles, now an old man (and looking more convincing as such than he does some 35 years later in *The Irishman*) replies – "No, it's just the way I see things." Leone and Noodles, like Pawnee in *The Revenant*, understand the emptiness of revenge. Bush, then Obama, then Trump might have learnt a lesson from them.

Once Upon a Time in Hollywood's reification of movie star culture and lust for violent revenge as a way of returning to the good old days, seems old-fashioned, tired and anachronistic – reactionary even. Tarantino set out to celebrate the late 1960s, a moment, half a century ago, similar to our own in so many ways. A moment where radical change is required and may now even be possible. As doyen of living Hollywood critics David Thompson goes on to say,

> *Once Upon a Time* is often a marvel of entertainment – Quentin is so talented – but in its violence, its regard for females and its curious unawareness of race, it demonstrates how far the fairy tales of Hollywood were from the realities of America by 2020.
>
> *(Thompson, 2020, p. 183)*

Through his revenge revisionism, his blind nostalgia, he trivialises history, politics and meaning so we can just "hang out". Films, as we have hopefully shown, are creations of their time and judged as such, but the way I see things today, at this time in American history, in his own words, I have to reject his hypothesis.

References

Black, J. (2019) '"You ain't gonna get away wit' this, Django": Fantasy, fiction and subversion in Quentin Tarantino's, Django Unchained'. *Quarterly Review of Film and Video.*

Chaney, J. (2019) On the Troubling Subtext of Once Upon a Time in Hollywood. *Vulture.* https://www.vulture.com/2019/08/once-upon-a-time-in-hollywood-and-its-troubling-subtext.html

Clark, S. and Mason, P. (eds.) (2015) *Macbeth. The Arden Shakespeare, third series.* London: Bloomsbury Publishing. Act 5, Scene 5.

Didion, J. (1968) *Slouching Toward Bethlehem*. Penguin.

Didion, J. (1979) *The White Album*. Penguin.

Hogeeven, E. (2020) 'Broad Horizons and Shallow Vistas in Chloé Zhao's *Nomadland*'. *Another Gaze.* https://www.anothergaze.com/broad-horizons-shallow-vistas-chloe-zhaos-nomadland-tiff-2020/

Marcuse, H. ([1964] 2002) *One-Dimensional Man*. London: Routledge Classics. Oxford Reference. https://www.oxfordreference.com/view/10.1093/oi/authority.20110803100416129

Marx, K. (1852) The Eighteenth Brumaire of Louis Bonaparte. *Internet Archive Wayback Machine*, http://www.marx2mao.com/M&E/EBLB52.html

Postman, N. (2006) *Amusing Ourselves to Death*. Penguin.

Pynchon, T. (1966) 'A Journey into the Mind of Watts'. *The New York Times*, June.

Pynchon, T. (2010) *Inherent Vice*. Vintage.

Suton, K. (2019) 'How Once Upon a Time in America became Leone's Butchered Swan Song'. *Beyond Cinephilia.* https://cinephiliabeyond.org/once-upon-a-time-in-america/.

Tallerico, B. (2019) https://www.rogerebert.com/reviews/once-upon-a-time-in–hollywood-2019.

Tarantino, Q. (2019) 'Shooting Star'. *The Spectator*, June. https://www.spectator.co.uk/article/shooting-star

Thompson, D. (2020) *A Light in the Dark: A History of Movie Directors.* W+N

Wassan, S. (2020) *The Big Goodbye: Chinatown and the Last Years of Hollywood.* Flatiron Books

CONCLUSION: REFLECTIONS ON THE USA PRESIDENTIAL ELECTIONS AND THE END OF TRUMP

The King is Dead; Long Live the King

The siege of the United States Capitol on 6 January 2021 vividly brings to mind Yeats's (1919) poem 'The Second Coming', "Things fall apart; the centre cannot hold; / Mere anarchy is loosed upon the world, / The blood-dimmed tide is loosed, and everywhere / The ceremony of innocence is drowned; / The best lack all conviction, while the worst / Are full of passionate intensity."

As with the films we have discussed, the reality behind the appearances is of a deeply divided, deeply tribalised, disunited state in which the idea of peaceful reconciliation, or any sort of an uncontested middle ground, has evaporated and the prospect of civil war in all but name haunts the streets.

If the American Dream represented a putative rallying cry, or place from which to build consensus, then all of that has been thrown into doubt. The deep divisions enacted by the films we have looked at are manifest in the current body politic, the schizoid body politic.

To see Trump as the problem is to ignore the deep divisions already manifest to these film-makers and represented across different social divisions: black and white (*Us*), rich and poor (*Joker*), the rule of law or the terrorist state (*Sicario*), male and female (*Widows*), educated and uneducated (*Roma*), indigenous peoples and their colonisers (*The Revenant*), all of which are the bastard children of the failed American Dream.

The bellwether of the American Dream is an idea of individual personal freedom that is precisely the deep motor of the current schisms. It is the refusal of the social, of the idea that we are all in this together, our deep dependence on each other and the current situation, that is reflected in the polls. It is personal responsibility versus social responsibility that is at the core of the problem.

But social responsibility gets rewritten as socialism, communism, dictatorship as opposed to solidarity, care, dependency and a recognition that there is

DOI: 10.4324/9781003206224-13

an alternative social order possible, one in which wider social needs can trump (pun intended) individual needs.

The liberal idea of individual freedom, at any cost, has taken over from any idea of even a modest social nature, despite the continuing advances in attachment theory and evolutionary biopsychology. Identity politics dominates the news, but the right to offend still takes precedent over the real systemic and institutional changes required.

At the deepest level, the survival of the planet as an ecologically sound going concern – no individual freedom can exist without it – requires that individuals are going to have to be constrained to do what is good for the whole system rather than their own myopic ends. This problematic is perfectly illustrated in *First Reformed*, even if the solution of individuals suddenly and improbably finding love for each other is no solution to the climate crisis.

As an origin story of the American Dream, *The Revenant* makes clear that the snake was already in the garden as the Indigenous peoples and their habitats are brutally and systematically destroyed for trinkets and trophies and whole civilisations are genocidally savaged.

What we are left with is damaged people acting as vigilantes to compensate in some measure for the systematic failures of the social order – as we see in *You Were Never Really Here* and *Joker*.

Meanwhile the futile attempts to deny history and tell a story with a happy ending – *Once Upon a Time in Hollywood* – are revealed as wish-fulfilling and illusory alternatives, denials, distractions and disavowals.

A similar though less strident dynamic is currently working its way out through the attempts to control the spread of coronavirus in the UK and the various forms of resistance to that, as we crash out of our relationship with the European Union, to our own social and economic detriment; a deliberate act of ideologically driven self-harm. Thus, the two long-term bastions of democracy in the West to date, the US and UK, are both hanging on at the ragged edge of democracy as the so-called 'popular vote' descends into rabid self-interest and schism.

I am reminded of the process of self-harm in which one part of the self, in order to rid itself of another hateful part of itself, feels forced to kill that part, forgetting that it is a part of itself. It turns out that Camus was probably right to signal that the problem of suicide is the "one truly serious philosophical problem" and that we need to recognise that "suicide is a permanent solution to a temporary problem."

Looking back at the self-harm done to the US by populist supporters of Trump, or at the economic and social damage in the UK that is still unfolding from the biblical approach to Brexit ("if thine eye offend thee, pluck it out, and cast it from thee") we must assume that there is a deep schism within these social orders, a polarisation that fetishises identity over community in a paradoxical way so that extreme nationalism and individualism are opposed to internationalism and community, even as Covid insists that 'we are all in this together'.

On the one hand, as Chris Hedges puts it in *The Great Delusion*,

> the real lesson we should learn from the rise of a demagogue such as Trump, who received 74 million votes, and a pandemic that our for-profit health care industry proved unable to contain, is that we are losing control as a nation and as a species. Far more dangerous demagogues will arise from the imperial and neoliberal policies the Biden administration will embrace. Far worse pandemics will sweep the globe with higher rates of infections and mortality, an inevitable result of our continued consumption of animals and animal products, and the wanton destruction of the ecosystem on which we and other species depend for life.
>
> *(Hedges, 2020)*

On the other hand, the Biden administration, in its approach to healthcare, climate policy and the economic stimulus package, has taken off at a sprint, in the most radical turnaround in American policy this century. Has the veteran of 50 years of politics learnt like the Silicon Valley culture that, in the age of surveillance capitalism, government must also 'move fast and mend things'?

The news from America? Signs of change, signs of hope, or just another temporary break from the trajectory of a dying middle class, a growing underclass, and a new neo-feudal digital billionaire class.

References

Hedges, C. (2021) The Great Delusion. https://scheerpost.com/2020/12/21/chris-hedges-the-great-delusion/

Yeats, W. B. (1919) *The Second Coming*. The Dial.

EPILOGUE: *NOMADLAND* (ZHAO, 2020)

Refuge of the Road: The Starry Misfits of Old New Frontiers

How They Came to California …

As we've seen in our introduction (particularly Churchwell (2021) and Adams (1931)) and via close analysis of *The Revenant*, America was built from a frontier mentality. From the Mayflower to the Alamo, the Europeans were searching for the next new place to conquer and harness nature. The continent was a huge space in which to do that, and in doing so, this mix of explorers, Puritans, rule-breakers, and risk-takers became Americans – wiping out the Indigenous tribes who had lived on the 'frontiers' for millennia in the process and then enslaving and forcibly shipping Black Africans across the Atlantic to work 'their' new land. De Tocqueville, James Baldwin, Ta-Nehesi Coates through the ages, have all spoken eloquently of the flaw in this American Dream, the original sin, and the need for reparation for these crimes that have continued into the twenty-first century.

How they then came to California is a story told in what many consider the best American film of this century in P. T. Anderson's *There Will be Blood*, and how the dream was built is told in Polanski's *Chinatown*, arguably the best film of America's 1970s cinematic renaissance. Both films tell the story of the corruption and unbridled greed that built the future of Los Angeles – "a bright and guilty place" according to Orson Welles, which for Mike Davis (1990) is "a stand in for capitalism in general … that has come to play the double role of utopia and dystopia for advanced capitalism" (Davis, 1990, p. 141). Davis's impassioned and in-depth analysis of the forces that shaped the city even in 1990 saw the significance of Towne's *Chinatown* and presciently Upton Sinclair's novel *Oil!* which was the inspiration for P. T. Anderson and Daniel Day Lewis's 2007 masterpiece.

DOI: 10.4324/9781003206224-14

Hollywood was built in the desert, created and irrigated by people like Noah Cross and Daniel Plainview – men that wanted to control the means of supply of water and oil, respectively. California had the perfect light for the studio system, and like all great frontiers, it had space. Space for white America's dreaming. The South Central of John Singleton's breakthrough *Boyz n the Hood* (1991), and the Watts that Pynchon (1966) watched burn in 1966, may as well have been another country to the white folk of Hollywood. As the *Los Angeles Times* (December 2001), in a report on the theft of black land, put it, "When they steal your land, they steal your future." Ta-Nehesi Coates in *The Case for Reparation* goes into the detail of the land grabs and segregations – "From the 1930s through the 1960s, black people across the country were largely and deliberately cut out of the legitimate home-mortgage market" (Coates, 2014).

In America in 2021, it is the past that is now most hotly contested. He who controls the narrative of the past can steal and control the future. It was Trump's thinly veiled vision of a return to a racist America that drove many of his supporters (consciously or not); revenge for the perceived ignominy of eight years of Obama. For every action there is an equal reaction, it seems, and for the last few years Hollywood has operated as a de facto opposition to Trump, championing its own diversity revolution through Me Too and Time's Up, with movie stars using the annual awards season to constantly speak up against the administration. The overall effect has seen each side become more and more entrenched in its own opinions, echo chambers and fake news. On the positive side at least, women's rights and diversity have won a number of battles to be finally seen and heard in Hollywood. In part, the structural changes that saw tech companies become studios has seen some shift in the old patriarchy. At the same time, it is no coincidence that the ability to challenge and cancel Weinstein et al. came at the very moment his power and that of the kingmakers of the independent world was waning, as 'Indiewood' was replaced or assimilated into the new streaming world order.

Outside of Hollywood, the new frontier of American life and discourse appears to be online. Clickbait and in-built bias, Russian troll factories, the data trawling and anti-privacy systems of surveillance capitalism have helped if not actually created this deep schism, this post-truth era. Democracy and the current iteration of the internet are uncomfortable bedfellows. The extreme binary nature and lack of nuance in Facebook, Twitter et al., mixed with an even greater primacy of the individual online, has seen the American Dream jettisoned for an American Nightmare of ever-deepening division.

Female Auteurs

As Trump was ejected from the White House, a film by a Chinese American woman, Chloe Zhao, came to dominate the 2021 awards season. Zhao had already made two powerful films – *Songs My Brother Taught Me* (2015) and

The Rider (2017) – both featuring and inspired by real people, both taking place on Native American Reservations, and both critically acclaimed. Her next film, *Nomadland*, was based on a non-fiction book about transient lifestyles in America after the 2008 crash (Bruder, 2017). A road movie of sorts, part epic poem to freewheeling America, part hybrid fiction, part circular descent into a Dante's Inferno of the American working poor.

The star of Zhao's *Nomadland*, Frances McDormand is a vocal and avowed feminist, Oscar-winner and liberal Hollywood icon. She embodies this unofficial opposition to Trump in Hollywood. She was one of only two professional actors in the film. The other was David Straithirn, a veteran of some six films by long-time campaigning left-wing activist writer / director John Sayles. Most of the featured cast were the real-life characters found in the book, including the real-life Bob Wells, who delivers the films big speech, about life, death and seeing each along the road. Wells is the figurehead of the 'Vandweller' movement and formed the Rubber Tramp Rendezvous, an annual gathering of the nomads, as featured in the film's denouement.

With *Nomadland, Variety* reported that, with "34 awards season trophies for directing, 13 for screenplay and nine for editing, Chloe Zhao has surpassed Alexander Payne (*Sideways*) as the most awarded person in a single awards season in the modern era."

This represents a significant step forward from the world described by New Queer Cinema Critic B. Ruby Rich in a scathing and prescient *Guardian* article, 'Get Your Dirty Hands Off Me', about male auteurs, and Orson Welles in particular. She describes a 'Women in Film' conference in 2003 where director Alison Anders,

> addressed the crisis facing women directors in both Hollywood and 'Indiewood'. The challenge, as always, was how to name the problem without sounding like a cry-baby or jinxing all future job prospects … Anders identified Welles as the source of their predicament. She pronounced the crowd to be suffering obvious symptoms of boy wonder syndrome: that is, the sorry state of being not-a-boy, and therefore not-a-wonder. Now, it was Welles himself who invented an alternative to being a Hollywood hack. The first conscious American auteur, Welles was determined to be his own man, beholden to no one.
>
> *(Ruby Rich, 2003)*

Rich's assertion that Welles was a conscious auteur is interesting, and to my mind wrongly conflates a distinct artistic vision with inherent sexism. Zhao's work after all clearly has such unity of vision, as do all of the female and diverse auteurs described herein. It is now possible, thankfully, for the 'girl wonder' to exist, and the three major Oscars this year went to female auteurs: to Zhao for *Nomadland* and to Emmerald Fennel for *Promising Young Woman*. Ironic too, given that Fincher's *Mank*, an origin story of sorts of

Citizen Kane, was one of the leading contenders to Zhao's *Nomadland* in awards season. Ruby Rich does clearly pinpoint the road American cinema has travelled and is on now – in the context of that 2003 article, it is somewhat encouraging that more women directors have started to make some real inroads into the miserly 7 per cent of American cinema they directed back then.

Misfits on the Old New Frontiers of *Nomadland*

Post-war America saw the emergence of the Beat Generation, most famously Kerouac's legendary American Road trip *On the Road* (1957) that defined a new generation. Bringing together for young white men the new world of "rock n roll youth culture" and a reboot of the eternal idea of the American frontier – an anthem for youth that inspired much culture, from iconic road movies like *Easy Rider* or *Thelma and Louise* to musicians as disparate as Bob Dylan and The Beastie Boys. For the Beats and Kerouac,

> the only people for me are the mad ones, the ones who are mad to live, mad to talk, mad to be saved, desirous of everything at the same time, the ones who never yawn or say a commonplace thing, but burn, burn, burn like fabulous yellow roman candles exploding like spiders across the stars and in the middle, you see the blue centerlight pop and everybody goes 'Awww!'
>
> *(Kerouac, 1957)*

The Misfits (1961) takes these mad ones and riffs off of the traditional western and *On the Road.* Arthur Miller had written a short story for *Esquire* entitled *Chicken Feed – The last Frontier of the Quixotic Cowboy* whilst waiting for his divorce to come through in Nevada in 1958. A few years later, he was on set filming it, with the legendary John Huston directing. Miller was already mid-divorce with his new wife Marilyn Monroe, for whom he had written the lead. Clark Gable was playing opposite her with Montgomery Clift and Eli Wallach.

Gable and Eli Wallach's broken cowboys, bent out of shape by war, ex-wives and economics, were clearly men out of time, reduced to capturing wild horses for pet food, and on a collision course with Monroe's animal-loving divorcee in the Nevada desert.

As William Reynolds, a self-proclaimed cowboy himself, brilliantly puts it,

> The West's place in that lineage was as a platform for expansion, discovery, and opportunity – a place where fortunes could be made as long as one held fast to pioneer spirit and grit and packed a gun. The movies of the time were not concerned with the resulting issues facing rangelands and those displaced by the forward thrust of an ever-engaging, Eastern-driven social and economic push for wealth and power.

> In the 1960s, the first Westerns set in the 20th century were produced. Reflecting the turbulence of the social climate of the '60s, Westerns became more and more politicized and concerned with the fallout of the rapid urbanization of the West and the effects it had on both people and the land. But the subject most '60s Western filmmakers seemed to depict loped around the perceived contradiction of the steadfast image of the cowboy trying to hang on in a modern world that seemed to be finished with him and his individualistic approach to life.
>
> *(Reynolds, 2006)*

Pauline Kael famously declared the western dead in 1974 – coincidentally the year that the New Hollywood peaked with Oscars for *Chinatown, The Conversation, The Godfather 2* and Gena Rowland's incredible performance in *A Woman Under the Influence.* At that same ceremony, as ever, the ghost at the table appeared in the shape of John Wayne, accepting an honorary award for John Ford's rival for the quintessential western director – Howard Hawks. Kael was right, the western never recovered fully, replaced as it was by the coming of the blockbuster via *Star Wars* and *Jaws*, but its influence still reverberates around the American psyche.

If timing is everything, *The Misfits* coincided with both the end of the popularity of the western, as highlighted and romanticised in Tarantino's *Once Upon a Time…* and the swan song of the studio system. Every year, the film has taken on more power and symbolic significance, not only but also because it was the last film for its two great stars. One who represented the old macho star system, the other who has stood in for every beautiful Hollywood starlet since. Monroe was sold for her sexual allure and abused by a system that rarely recognised or celebrated her undoubted intelligence and talent.

The terrifying, cruel and gruelling horse capture sequence (it would never have been allowed on-set in today's world of animal rights), shot in the last few days of production, almost certainly contributed to Clark Gable's death ten days later. Gable collapsed with a heart attack the day after wrap and never recovered. Less than a year later, Marilyn Monroe died alone in suspicious circumstances, taking the secrets of presidents and playwrights to her grave. Montgomery Clift too, after his car crash of 1956, was a shadow of the star he had been, and this was his last great movie. Only Wallach would survive the film and return to help reinvent the western in one of Leone's spaghetti reboots of the genre *The Good, The Bad and the Ugly.* John Huston would go on to make *Fat City* (1972) and *The Dead* (1987) – with daughter Anjelica, and more significantly star alongside his daughter's long-time boyfriend Jack Nicholson in *Chinatown.* As the BFI's Geoff Andrew put it – "The Misfits is the film that fate helped make a classic" (Andrews, 2015).

If *The Misfits* shows us that the battle for the West is still one between man and nature, or more specifically man's relationship to nature and the economy, it also points at two aspects of the crisis of the American Dream and capitalism that Zhao returns to in *Nomadland* – our place in the universe and the decline of the family. The link across 60 years of Hollywood history is in a scene from each film that replicates the other. The fucked-up family by the Nevada desert campfire, out hunting horses for dogfood in *The Misfits*, becomes Frances McDormand's Fern with Straithirn's Dave in an iconic National Park looking up at the stars.

It's Wonderful to Know Things

During the star-gazing scene in *Nomadland*, a park guide describes the stars to a group that Dave and Fern are with. He points to Vega and tells them that it is 24 light years away and that the light they are seeing left Vega in 1987 and has only just got here. He continues by telling them that plasma from stars hits the Earth's soil and becomes a part of us. As Joni Mitchell sings in "Woodstock" (Mitchell, 1970) and Zhao seems to be suggesting throughout, we are made from stardust, and there is a felt need to get ourselves back to the garden of Eden.

Similarly, in *The Misfits* Wallach's character, Guido, desperate to woo Monroe's Roslyn from under the nose of Gable's Gay, discusses the heavens around their last campfire together, telling Roslyn that the star he is pointing to is so far away that by the time its light reaches them, it might not be there anymore. Roslyn replies, without irony, that it is "wonderful to know things", while Gay quips that "us ignorant folk" have to hit the hay.

But up there in the desert, away from their makeshift half-built home, all is revealed. Even their dog senses things are off, on a precipice. Guido tells Roslyn, when she asks why the dog shakes, that it isn't the horses that the dogs are frightened of but the humans. Dogs were wild once, and when the dog is reminded of this, it is scared that they are going to end up dead too.

Later, after a huge struggle capturing the wild horses, Gay, broken in every way as a cowboy, releases them at Roslyn's hysterical request. When the two are alone again on the road back to Reno, in the last scene either of these great actors will ever appear in, Roslyn seems to tell Gay it's over between them. They stop the car, and Gay watches her pick up the dog from the camp and says "God bless you girl." Roslyn, like Fern, is clearly allied with nature, she loves all living things. Roslyn, responding to Gay's proposal earlier in the film to have children together, tells him that she was scared at the beginning, but that she is not so scared now. She pauses and speaks the last line of her career, enquiring: "How do you find your way back in the dark?" Gay grasps at Roslyn's words. Like Peter Pan's advice to Wendy to take the second star on the right, he suggests that she heads for the big star straight on, where she will find the highway under it to take them right home.

Some see the stars as new frontier. In cinema during the Trump era, we witnessed the heroism of Gosling's Armstrong in the underrated *First Man* and the *Heart of Darkness*-like *Ad Astra*. Madness and obsession drive both these frontiersmen. At the same time, the new Silicon Valley billionaire class turn to the new American frontier of space exploration, abandoned by government not long after the Challenger disaster and now taken up by the two wealthiest men on the planet – Jeff Bezos and Elon Musk. Of course, *Nomadland* uses an Amazon depot to portray the precarity and soullessness of modern work. So, it is with some sad irony that 'we the people' must witness this affront to the nation – a start-up space race – completely out of step with nature again. Amazon (and the other tech companies) conquer and commodify every area of our daily life whilst vastly underpaying both their taxes and their own workers. They then spend the profits accrued on vanity projects inspired by Captain Kirk's 1960s "space, the final frontier" dream. Gil Scott-Heron, in his song 'Whitey on the Moon' of 1970, showed the bitter irony of being unable to afford the doctor's bill when a rat bites his sister in their impoverished housing, while 'Whitey's on the moon', as true today but still lost on Bezos and Musk it seems.

Uncharted Territories of the American Family

Sarah Connors comments in *Terminator 2* that the future had been clear to her, but it is now like a dark highway at night and that they are in uncharted territory and making it up as they go along. As the end of the old century approached, for the splintering American Family, Connors words rang truer than ever.

Like *Back to the Future*, truly the great reactionary franchise of the Reagan era (a fantasy that only by returning to the 1950s can we save the family / future), or a good ol' John Wayne movie, Trump would have had us return to a time that never fully existed – the post-war white enclaves and picket fences of a small-town America with perfect nuclear families eating together, then hiding under tables from the Communist Red threat of Armageddon. The family ship was already sailing in 1980s American culture, despite Nancy and Ronnie's best efforts. As picked apart already in 1986 by David Lynch in *Blue Velvet*, even this idealised utopia had its dark secrets. But as the 1950s fell away, the *Misfits* stared down the barrel of the gun that was divorce and displacement American style. We meet Monroe and Gable's characters at the end of marriages. Gay we see is estranged, mocked even by his now grown-up children, in a painful sequence at a Reno bar. Rising divorce rates, sexual liberty, atomisation, and individual freedoms began to take their toll on the imperfect model of American patriarchal family and its 2.4 kids. *The Misfits* reflects these broken ideals, as the four protagonists form a strange, fucked-up family of sorts around a campfire in the desert.

Some 30 years on, Fred Pfeil's essay 'Home Fires Burning, Family Noir in *Blue Velvet* and *Terminator 2*' describes how

> home and family are being destabilized, noir-ized in both. The large differences between these two films, in terms of aesthetic strategies and

> audiences, only make the similarities of results of each film's processing of *noir* elements that much more striking and significant.
>
> ...
>
> This relocation of the family unit of Mommy/Daddy/Baby to the place where the noir hero used to be, out in public and on the run, is likewise braided with a complex transfiguration of all three roles in the family romance, part transforming and part regressive in each case. Most prominently is of course ultra-buff Linda Hamilton's Sarah Conner as fully operational warrior-woman, like Sigourney Weaver's Ripley in Cameron's *Aliens* only more so, phallic mother with a complete set of soldier-of-fortune contacts, cache of weapons and survivalist skills. Conversely, there is 'the Arnold', fresh from *Kindergarten Cop* and therefore all the more available for refunctioning from killing machine to nurturant proto-father who, as Sarah's own voice-over puts it, "*would always be there and would always protect him i.e., John the son. Of all the would-be fathers, this machine was the only one that measured up.*" And finally, rounding out this new holy family is golden-boy John, who as grown-up rebel leader sends Arnold back to the past to protect his childhood self, but who as a kid must teach both Mom and Dad how and when to cool their jets.
>
> *(Pfeil, 1993, pp. 227, 244)*

In *The Misfits*, the family is destroyed like the cowboy way of life, children are dislocated, absent. Thirty years on, still in the desert and on the road, the future in *Terminator 2* can only be saved by a father who is "more human than human", a mother who is a 'can do it all' warrior and a child that is essentially parent to himself.

In *Nomadland*, Fern and Dave stand with a huge dinosaur at a roadstop attraction (a symbol of humanity's own precarious state during the Anthropocene). I last remember this Brontosaurus on screen in another outsider's view of the mythic West, Wim Wenders' – *Paris, Texas* (1983). Sam Shepherd's Travis (Harry Dean Stanton), his son Hunter and his estranged wife Jane (Natassia Kinski), like the main characters in *The Misfits, Blue Velvet* and *Terminator 2*, form another impossible family. By the end of the film we realise, despite Travis's odyssey, they can never be reunited – always seen as a combination of two in the film, they are only a whole three in a memorable cine-film sequence that compels the broken Travis to act. They could even be how Roslyn and Gay from *The Misfits* might turn out if they did make a go of it and have a kid. Tragically, Travis at the end of *Paris, Texas* seems destined to leave his family behind and re-enter his own Nomadland.

In what could easily be a description of *Nomadland*, Sven Mikulek writes of *Paris, Texas* in his article for the wonderful *Cinephilia and Beyond*:

> It has an economy of the visually enticing road film that centers far more on emotion that action, that leans on subtlety and the inner world of its

> heroes… As a poetic exploration of character set against the grandiose mythological background of Western America … and with such passion and reverence that could only come from an eye and artistic soul of a foreigner. What many people immediately associate with the film, however, is its visual identity. Breathtaking shots … bathed in sunlight, decorated with lonesome gas stations, steaming roads that cut through the brown, dusty carpet that stretches far towards the ocean, lost people trying to find their place under the scorching sun… a script that allows the viewers to be gently sucked in the atmosphere and swept by the power of the scarcely uttered words.
>
> *(Mikulek, 2018)*

The Misfits, Paris, Texas, Nomadland – this triptych of westerns without cowboys across the last 60 years show us the fate of the family in America. The family is an impossible dream. *Nomadland* skirts around the hard issues of late capitalism, as we shall see, but Fern's damaged, lonely character represents the end point for the disintegrating family in this society.

The Refuge of the Road

In Joni Mitchell's "Refuge of the Road", all the romance of the road movie, or the road novel, *On the Road* for instance, are condensed into a perfect song about the joys and excitement of being on the road and its attendant hardships. Going for refuge is also coincidentally a phrase to describe a Buddhist approach to seeking enlightenment as a way of protecting ourselves from danger and at the same time safeguarding what is most valuable and beautiful within us.

In *Nomadland*, Fern is widowed and living out of a van. She rejects the offer of home comforts from a man, Dave, who she meets on the road and later from her sister too. Both explicitly ask her to stay in their beautiful family homes. She makes a clear choice at key moments in the film that what family life she ever had ended with her husband's death, and the voiceover featuring Shakespeare's Sonnet 18, harking back to her wedding vows as a young woman, seems to underline she can only manage the loss by moving ever on.:

> Nor shall Death brag thou wander'st in his shade, When in eternal lines to time thou grow'st; So long as men can breathe or eyes can see, So long lives this, and this gives life to thee

She has been nomadic since losing her husband Beau, and the town where they lived, Empire, Nevada lost its main source of employment – a Gypsum plant. She has no future, and she trawls a circular route on the road. No youthful upstart Dean Moriarty, she's of retirement age but lives in a kind of voluntary discomfort, partially forced upon her by the limits of well-paid work – the seasonal low-paid Amazon depot that she works at every Christmas – and partly by the collapsed economy of her hometown. She also explicitly rejects mainstream society's comforts, offered to her at various points, in favour of the open road, gorgeous vistas and nature's horizons. The discomforts of shitting in a bucket, working in precarious 'McJobs' and dealing with broken down vans, for Fern, are outweighed by the nomadic lifestyle and communing with nature's elements. Water, as in *Roma* and *The Revenant*, cleanses and carries her, whilst the sun always sets in the West. It is clear that in grief Fern has chosen the "refuge of the road", and in my mind, Joni Mitchell's song resonates throughout. She is constantly drifting and leaving, unable to settle even when good opportunities arise. Throughout, Zhao frames her alone in shot, dwarfed by huge vistas, and often separate from people.

Despite critical acclaim in the mainstream, Zhao was criticised by her adaptation of the more overtly political book in an essay – 'The Neoliberal Fantasy at the Heart of "Nomadland"' (Gupta, 2021):

> Bruder took to the highway as well, in a white van named Halen. She profiled 'nomads' – some who play themselves in the film – reduced to living out of vehicles after losing jobs, savings, homes. They faced 'impossible choices': food or dental work, mortgage or electric bill, car payment or medicine. But they embraced the minimalist lifestyle: 'You have a choice – you can be free, or you can be homeless,' says one.
>
> Fern doesn't struggle with injury or illness or fatigue or shame. Most of her time is leisure, not labor: makeshift spas, wildlife tours, park hikes, campfires, star watching. The cost of working the sugar-beet harvest in Nebraska is the dirt washing off Fern's neck. The reality for Bruder, 'in reasonably good shape' in her thirties, was harsher. Of her first full shift, she writes, 'My whole body hurt.' Injuries were common. Most workers quit. The film does show Linda May, a real-life nomad who plays herself, confronting impossible options. Faced with living on $550 a month, she considers suicide by booze and propane stove. But the many tales of monetary woes in Bruder's book are otherwise ignored.

It is true that the heart of the original book is largely rejected for a romanticised version of the lifestyle in the film. Even the conditions at the Amazon depot are underplayed. It would be hard to imagine a world in which the behemoth company would allow one of its workers to declare onscreen that the company was "probably the biggest slave owner in the world" (Bruder, 2017) and still give Zhao permission to film inside. Amazon is the epitome of capitalist realism at work – on the surface and for its customers the biggest superstore in the world, with shiny goods arriving miraculously at your door in hours. A service that, of course, massively increased in value during the strange days of lockdown, but for its factory workers, drivers and vendors was a far more painful proposition. In cinema, Ken Loach's *Sorry, We Missed You* (2019) deals a sharper body blow to the Amazon myth of a fast frictionless service.

Despite her significant breakthrough for women and minorities in the award season, Zhao's film is accused of foregrounding Fern at the expense of the clear context of post-2008 crash America.

> The distracting vistas, combined with the fact that Fern and her contemporaries are all essentially good humoured, non-threatening, and uncomplaining, make us almost forget that they are seeking alternative ways to live because their government has left them lacking homes, healthcare, or other forms of social safety, and that this could very reasonably inspire resentment....
>
> Zhao strives to spotlight a protagonist making space for possibilities within a limited range of options; however, in overemphasising the beauty of Fern's resilience and the views from her dashboard, the filmmaker regrettably occludes both a sense of depth and the essential messiness of context.
>
> *(Hogeveen, 2020)*

As a filmmaker, Zhao, like all of us, walks a tightrope between critique and collaboration with the ubiquity of the system, but as she herself puts it,

> I tried to focus on the human experience and things that I feel go beyond political statements to be more universal – the loss of a loved one, searching for home ... I keep thinking about my family back in China – how would they feel about a cowboy in South Dakota, or a woman in her 60s living in America? ... If I make it too specific to any issues, I know it's going to create a barrier. They'd go, 'That's their problem.'
>
> *(Marchetti, 2021)*

The style that Zhao developed over three films is a hybrid of poetic drama and documentary realism – she is on the edge of both, a beautifully singular voice with antecedents in Robert Altman, Errol Morris, Sarah Polley's *Stories We Tell* (2012) and Bart Layton's *The Imposter* (2012) and *American Animals* (2018). *Nomadland*'s main character also chimes with two Portland-based films *Pig* (2020) and *Leave No Trace* (2018) that beautifully track men who retreat from modern America into the wilderness to avoid the pain of loss.

Zhao's work is a crossing point between fact and fiction that mirrors our post-truth world.

It is also a difficult crossing point between the two superpowers of the twenty-first century – America and China. Hollywood desperately needs Chinese box office, but for the first time since 1969, the Chinese authorities did not show the Oscars, and during her awards run, Beijing-born, middle-class Zhao "was made *persona non gratis* in her home country" (Davis, 2021).

B. Ruby Rich commissioned Chinese cinema expert Gina Marchetti to write an intricate piece about *Nomadland* and Zhao's relationship to China, which concludes:

> References to China in *Nomadland* remain oblique, seen only through the goods distributed via the Amazon warehouse, but these indirect connections do allow viewers to glimpse the consequences of global capitalism on screen. Zhao leaves the rest to her audiences to piece together. The director remains careful, for a reason: surely, she hopes to show her films (including Marvel's *The Eternals*, currently in production) back in China. Minority unrest, border politics, land rights, and labor unions are subjects which, even if confined to the American West, may go too far, under current circumstances. Zhao knows the rules but, given China's reaction to her historic Oscar win, that may no longer be good enough.
>
> *(Marchetti, 2021)*

Even more revelatory of her auteur intentions, (un)conscious desires, before *Nomadland* was even made, Zhao said in an interview:

> I'm an only child, and I love being on my own. I love being completely independent. But my parents are getting older, I've got two dogs, and suddenly, I can't live without them… As a human being, you're constantly trying to see how much you're willing to be part of a community, and how much you want to be on your own. I think about that all the time, and I struggle with that.
>
> *(Lazic, 2018)*

Nomadland and Zhao's focus is clearly Fern, not the system that created her. Her journey through grief is a lonely, circular one, and without judgement Zhao beautifully portrays a simple, singular life. Transcendence, the sea, the sky, the forests are what interest her. Her next film for Marvel, *The Eternals* portrays an ancient immortal hidden race amongst us who will rescue mankind in its hour of need. But here on Earth, no one is coming, and we have to save ourselves. It's too late to go back to the garden, the old way of life of the Native Americans. The light of dying stars reflects back upon us, but if we continue to completely ignore our natural environment, we will soon go the same way of the stars.

More precarious still than Fern are those who live literally and figuratively on the roadside, the street and in the gutter – the near million of the Skid Rows of America are the nations invisible dispossessed. They are also predominantly ethnic minorities. Those portrayed in *Nomadland* are the new white misfits. In Zhao's portrayal, these dispossessed are not so much given no choice, but consider themselves happier with this transient chance to be in nature and to keep moving. Perhaps the reality of life on the road is much harsher, but that is clearly not Zhao's preoccupation here.

In the film's climax, by a campfire again, Bob and his van friends gather to pay tribute to one they have lost. The morning after, Bob speaks warmly to Fern. For the first time she opens up, revealing that she never had kids, and that, when her husband died, she couldn't move on. She remembers her father and his saying that "what is remembered remains", and then that perhaps she spent too much time remembering.

Bob tells her that he can relate to what she is saying, and that he rarely talks about his son who five years ago took his own life. For a long hard time, he couldn't confront that fact without asking himself why he didn't kill himself. But he came to realise that he could honour his son by helping and serving people, and sometimes that is all he has, to keep going. One thing he loves about the nomad life is the illusion that there are no final goodbyes: "I always just say, 'I'll see you down the road.' And I do."

In America if you are not at home, you are "on the road" like your forefathers – Glass and Fitzgerald in *The Revenant* or Daniel Boone. In Cormac McCarthy's father and son parable *The Road* (2006), Jack Kerouac's dream and James Cameron's nightmare finds its terminus – it is the road inverted. *The Road* is a search for some hope of life at the end of the world, but as ever a journey taken west in search of a frontier of survival and sustenance. It ends in uncertainty with a boy on the shore at the edge of the world, orphaned. The family is gone – three is no longer the magic number.

In this new America of broken families, or worse still individuals who cannot exist within relationships, the road is not just freedom, it may also be a place to be lost or disassociate from loss – to literally lose oneself. We return with *Nomadland* to a cinema of loneliness.

A State of Sedimentation; a State of Separation

We began this journey because we love cinema, we loved the communal nature of the big screen palaces, the films projected onto the wall of Plato's Cave, being alone and yet together in the dark. Globalisation has rendered divisions between us wider, not brought us together. The world over the last five years appears to have moved into smaller communities, and the communal, common moment is hard to find. Our opinions have become sedimentary, stuck. We have retreated into our homes to consume visual content partly by choice, partly by necessity under conditions of a global pandemic. More than ever, we consume cinema online and alone.

As Bo Burnham, pioneer YouTuber turned writer / director / stand-up / singer, asks with some irony in what may be the defining art piece of the pandemic, "Inside"

> Is it necessary that every single person on this planet, um, expresses every single opinion that they have on every single thing, that occurs all at the same time? Is that … Is that necessary? Or to ask in a different way, can anyone … anyone shut the fuck up … about anything? About any single thing for an hour? And I know you're thinking you're not shutting the fuck up now … but … (cuts to next song).
>
> *(Burnham, 2021)*

At the same time, the US Marines recruits by acknowledging American youth's struggle with the ever-present online world by releasing a promotional video 'Battle to Belong':

> Some of what you seek can be found online, but for Marines, the things that matter most must be fought for: a true sense of purpose that comes from knowing you are part of something bigger than yourself.
>
> *(US Marines, 2021)*

How do we unpick a world where loneliness and confusion on the internet is the rallying call for both liberal insiders and the US military?

A Way in the Dark

In the strictly binary state of Trump's America, where 70 million people still voted for a man who had failed them at the greatest moment of crisis, we understand clearly that the American Dream is broken. Democracy is in crisis. The primacy of the individual over the society and all the attendant problems of such atomisation outlined serves very few of us. The architecture of the internet and the final frontier of commodification – of us – deepens our divisions, isolates us all further.

Where we began this book with Glass and his not so merry band destroying the Indian Nation, we end it with Fern on the road. A more natural world. One with which America is clearly out of step.

We are back where we began. A circular route, in the beginning is our end. There is no real refuge in the road or the stars or alone. We have just the one planet. And each other to find a way in the dark.

> Our lives are communal, and without others we would languish and die. Personal relations are the essence of our existence. In addition also without personal relations there would be no person which sounds somewhat paradoxical until we realise that we are adapted to looking for and sustaining just such personal relationships from birth, … later because we have a relationship with the society and culture of a village, town … and country which can develop into a relationship with a wider community which is predicated upon having become a personal being first. Our lives

> are our lives in common despite our desperate need to believe in the complete authorship of our own individuality. Our individuality only makes sense in a specific and cultural social context.
>
> *(Clarke, 2006)*

References

Adams, J. T. (1931 [2017]) *The Epic of America*. New York: Routledge.

Andrews, G. (2015) 'The film that fate helped made a classic: The Misfits'. *BFI*. https://www2.bfi.org.uk/news-opinion/news-bfi/features/film-fate-helped-make-classic-misfits

Bruder, J. (2017) *Nomadland*. W.W. Norton and Co.

Burnham, B. (2021) *Bo Burnham: Inside*. Netflix.

Churchwell, S. (2021) 'A Brief History of the American Dream '. *The Catalyst*, 21 (Winter).

Clarke, G. S. (2006) *Personal Relations Theory: Fairbairn, Macmurray and Suttie*. London: Routledge.

Coates, T.-N. (2014) 'The Case for Reparations'. *The Atlantic*. https://www.theatlantic.com/magazine/archive/2014/06/the-case-for-reparations/361631/

Davis, M. (1990) *City of Quartz: Excavating the Future in Los Angeles*. Haymarket

Davis, R. (2021) 'Nomadland censored by China after Nationalist Backlash'. *Variety* (March). https://variety.com/2021/film/news/chloe-zhao-nomadland-china-censorship-1234922882/?fbclid=IwAR2wm2pZDMM3rt-XYHnGbSbDzUwqharM5idjjI6vlZb_Dm_Xi2LpZH2GGUA

Gupta, F. (2021) 'The Neoliberal Fantasy at the Heart of "Nomadland" '. *In these times.com*. https://inthesetimes.com/article/nomadland-chloe-zhao-oscars-film-culture-amazon-workers

Hogeveen, E. (2020) 'Broad Horizons and Shallow Vistas in Chloé Zhao's "Nomadland"'. *Another Gaze* (September). https://www.anothergaze.com/broad-horizons-shallow-vistas-chloe-zhaos-nomadland-tiff-2020/

Kerouac, J. (1957) *On the Road*. New York: Viking Press.

Lazic, E. (2018) 'Interview: Chloé Zhao on *The Rider*, her feminist film about masculinity'. *Seventh Row*. https://seventh-row.com/2018/04/27/chloe-zhao-rider

Lewan, T. and Barclay, D. (2001) 'When they steal your land, they steal your future'. *LA Times*. https://www.latimes.com/archives/la-xpm-2001-dec-02-mn-10514-story.html

Marchetti, G. (2021) 'Chloé Zhao and China: The *Nomadland* Moment'. *Film Quarterly*. https://filmquarterly.org/2021/04/28/chloe-zhao-and-china-the-nomadland-moment/

Mikulec, S. (2018) '"Paris, Texas": Wim Wenders' Film of Extraordinary Beauty and Irresistibility'. *Cinephilia and Beyond*. https://cinephiliabeyond.org/paris-texas-wim-wenders-film-extraordinary-beauty-irresistibility/

Pfeil, F. (1993) 'Home Fires Burning, Family Noir in *Blue Velvet* and *Terminator 2*'. In J. Copjec (ed.), *Shades of Noir: A Reader*. London and New York: Verso.

Pynchon, T. (1966) 'A Journey into the Mind of Watts'. *The New York Times*.

Reynolds, W. (2006) 'The Misfits'. *Cowboys and Indians*. http://www.wcreynolds.com/images/writings/Film_MISFITS.pdf.

Ruby Rich, B. (2003) 'Get Your Dirty Hands Off Me'. *The Guardian*. https://www.theguardian.com/film/2003/aug/29/1

US Marines (2020) 'Battle to Belong '. *Youtube*. Online advert. https://www.youtube.com/watch?v=bCjEV75F2tM

FILMOGRAPHY

Featured Films (in Chapter Order)

The Revenant (2015) Iñárritu, A. G. USA
Roma (2018) Cuarón, A. USA / Mex
First Reformed (2017) Schrader, P. USA
Sicario (2015) Villeneuve, D. USA
Joker (2019) Phillips, T. USA
You Were Never Really Here (2017) Ramsay, L. USA / Fr
Widows (2018) McQueen, S. USA
Us (2019) Peele, J. USA
Once Upon a Time in Hollywood (2019) Tarantino, Q. USA
Nomadland (2020) Zhao, C. USA

Other Films by Chapter / Alphabetical Order of Film Title

Chapter 1 External Worlds

Adaptation (2002) Kaufman, C. USA
Bonnie and Clyde (1967) Penn, A. USA
Dirty Harry (1971) Siegel, D. USA
Easy Rider (1969) Hopper, D. USA
Marriage Story (2019) Baumbach, N. USA
Medium Cool (1969) Wexler, H. USA
The French Connection (1971) Friedkin, W. USA
The Great Hack (2019), Noujaim, J. and Amera, K. USA
The Irishman (2019) Scorsese, M. USA
Teenager vs Superpower (2017) Piscatella, J. Hong Kong

DOI: 10.4324/9781003206224-15

TV / Series

Can't Get You Out of My Head, (2021) Curtis, A. UK
Chernobyl (2019) Mazin, C. UK
The Power of Nightmares (2004) Curtis, A. UK
Top of the Lake (2013) Campion, J. Aus / USA
Too Old to Die Young (2019) Refn, N.W. USA
True Detective (2014) Pizzolatto, N. USA

Chapter 2 Internal Worlds

Alien (1979) Scott, R. USA
Ocean's Eleven (2001) Soderbergh, S. USA
The Dirty Dozen (1967) Aldrich, R. USA
The Seven Samurai (1954) Kurosawa, A. Japan
X-Men (2000) Singer, B. USA

Chapter 3 The Revenant

Biutiful (2013) Iñárritu, A. G. Spain

Chapter 4 Roma

Ben Hur (1959) Wyler, W. USA
Bicycle Thieves (1948) De Sica, V. Italy
Carne y arena (Flesh and Sand – 2017) Iñárritu, A. G. Mexico
Children of Men (2006) Cuarón, A. UK / USA
Gravity (2013) Cuarón, A. USA
Rome, Open City (1945) Rossellini, R. USA
The Road to Roma (2020) Clariond, A. and Nuncio, G. USA / Mex.
Y tu mamá también (2001) Cuarón, A. Mexico

Chapter 5 First Reformed

American Gigolo (1980) Schrader, P. USA
Apocalypse Now (1979) Coppola, F. F. USA
A Quiet Place (2018) Krasinski, J. USA
Avengers – Endgame, (2019) The Russo Bros. USA
Blade Runner (1982) Scott, R. USA
Chinatown (1974) Polanski, R. USA
Elysium (2013) Blomkamp, N. USA
ET (1982) Spielberg, S. USA
I am Legend (2007) Lawrence, F. USA
Interstellar (2014) Nolan, C. USA

Jaws (1975) Spielberg, S. USA
Joker (2019) Philips, T. USA
M (1931) Lang, M. USA
Mad Max: Fury Road (2015) Miller, G. Aus / USA
Mean Streets (1973) Scorsese, M. USA
Nashville (1975) Altman, R. USA
Once Upon a Time in Hollywood (2019) Tarantino, Q. USA
Planet of the Apes (1968) Schaffner, F. USA
Raging Bull (1980) Scorsese, M. USA
Raiders of the Lost Ark (1981) Spielberg, S. USA
Stalker (1979) Tarkovsky, A. USSR
Star Wars (1977) Lucas, G. USA
Taxi Driver (1976) Scorsese, M. USA
The Conversation (1974) Coppola, F. F. USA
The Day After (1983) Meyer, N. USA
The Godfather (1972) Coppola, F. F. USA
The Irishman (2019) Scorsese, M. USA
The Midnight Sky (2020) Clooney, G. USA
The Road (2009) Hillcoat, J. USA
Wall-E (2008) Stanton, A. USA
World War Z (2013) Foster, M. USA
You Were Never Really Here (2017) Ramsay, L. USA / Fr

Chapter 6 Sicario

Arrival (2016) Villeneuve, D. USA
Blade Runner 2049 (2017) Villeneuve, D. USA
Blue Velvet (1986) Lynch, D. USA
Chinatown (1974) Polanski, R. USA
Dog Day Afternoon (1975) Lumet, S. USA
Dune (2021) Villeneuve, D. USA
Enemy (2013) Villeneuve, D. USA
ET (1982) Spielberg, S. USA
Green Zone (2010) Greengrass, P. USA
Hell or High Water (2016) Mackenzie, D. USA
Incendies (2010) Villeneuve, D. Canada
Prisoners (2013) Villeneuve, D. USA
Rendition (2007) Hood, G. USA
Seven (1995) Fincher, D. USA
Sicario 2: Day of the Soldado (2018) Sollima, S. USA
The Hurt Locker (2008) Bigelow, K. USA
The Silence of the Lambs (1991) Demme, J. USA
Wind River (2017) Sheridan, T. USA
Zero Dark Thirty (2012) Bigelow, K. USA

Chapter 7 Joker

Aquaman (2018) Wan, J. USA
Black Panther (2018) Coogler, R. USA
Dressed To Kill (1980) De Palma, B. USA
Iron Man (2008) Favreau, J. USA
Superman – Man of Steel (2013) Snyder, Z. USA
The Dark Knight (2008) Nolan, C. USA
The King of Comedy (1982) Scorsese, M. USA
The Master (2012) Anderson P. T. USA
Thor: Ragnorak (2017) Waititi, T. USA
Vertigo (1958) Hitchcock, A. USA
Wonder Woman (2017) Jenkins, P. USA

TV / Series

The Mandalorian (2019) Favreau, J. Disney+
WandaVision (2021) Shakman, M. Disney+

Chapter 8 You Were Never Really Here

Morvern Callar (2002) Ramsay, L. UK
Psycho (1960) Hitchcock, A. USA
Ratcatcher (1999) Ramsay, L. UK
The Shawshank Redemption (1994) Darabont, F. USA
We Need to Talk about Kevin (2011) Ramsay, L. UK

Chapter 9 Widows

Boogie Nights (1997) Anderson, P. T. USA
Casablanca (1942) Curtiz, M. USA
Dog Day Afternoon (1975) Lumet, S. USA
Gone Girl (2014) Fincher, D. USA
Heat (1995) Mann, M. USA
Hunger (2008) McQueen, S. UK
Magnolia (1999) Anderson, P. T. USA
Nashville (1975) Altman, R. USA
Ocean's 8 (2018) Ross, G. USA
Set It Off (1996) F Gary Gray. USA
Shame (2011) McQueen, S. UK
Short Cuts (1993) Altman, R. USA
Silver City (2004) Sayles, J. USA
Sunshine State (2002) Sayles, J. USA
12 Years a Slave (2013) McQueen, S. USA

Thelma and Louise (1991) Scott, R. USA
The Usual Suspects (1995) Singer, B. USA

TV / Series

Lovers Rock (2020) McQueen, S. UK
Prime Suspect (1992) La Plante, L. UK
The Wire (2002–2008) Chase, D. USA

Chapter 10 Us

Carrie (1976) De Palma, B. USA
Crash (2004) Haggis, P. USA
Get Out (2017) Peele, J. USA
Green Book (2018) Farrelly, P. USA
Parasite (2019) Joon-Ho, B. South Korea
Rosemary's Baby (1968), Polanski, R. USA
Shoplifters (2018) Koreeda, H. Japan
The Exorcist (1973) Friedkin, W. USA
The Shining (1980) Kubrick, S. USA / UK
Them! (1954) Gordon, D. USA
They Live (1988) Carpenter, J. USA

TV / Series

Lovecraft Country (2020) Green, M. USA
The Twilight Zone (2019) Peele, J. USA

Chapter 11 Once Upon a Time in Hollywood

Django Unchained (2012) Tarantino, Q. USA
Inglorious Bastards (2009) Tarantino, Q. USA
Inherent Vice (2014) Anderson, P. T. USA
Jackie Brown (1997) Tarantino, Q. USA
Kill Bill (2003) Tarantino, Q. USA
Mulholland Drive (2001) Lynch, D. USA
Once Upon a Time in America (1984) Leone, S. USA
Once Upon a Time in the West (1968) Leone, S. USA / Italy
Pulp Fiction (1994) Tarantino, Q. USA
Reservoir Dogs (1991) Tarantino, Q. USA
Rosemary's Baby (1968) Polanski, R. USA
The Godfather (1972) Coppola, F. F. USA
The Hateful Eight (2015) Tarantino, Q. USA
True Romance (1993) Scott, T. USA

Conclusion and Epilogue

A Woman Under the Influence (1974) Cassavetes, J. USA
Ad Astra (2019) Gray, J. USA
Aliens (1986) Cameron, J. USA
American Animals (2018) Layton, B. USA
Blue Velvet (1986) Lynch, D. USA
Boyz n the Hood (1991) Singleton, J. USA
Chinatown (1974) Polanski, R. USA
Citizen Kane (1941) Welles, O. USA
Fat City (1972) Huston, J. USA
First Man (2018) Chazelle, D. USA
Inside (2021) Burnham, B. USA
Jaws (1975) Spielberg, S. USA.
Kindergarten Cop (1990) Reitman, I. USA
Leave No Trace (2018) Granik, D. USA
Mank (2020) Fincher, D. USA
Nomadland (2020) Zhao, C. USA
Paris, Texas (1984) Wenders, W. USA
Pig (2021), Sanoski, M USA
Promising Young Woman (2020) Fennell, E. USA
Songs My Brothers Taught Me (2015) Zhao, C. USA
Star Wars (1977) Lucas, G. USA
Sorry we missed you (2019) Loach, K. USA
Stories we tell (2012) Polley, S.
Terminator 2 (1991) Cameron, J. USA
The Revenant (2015) Iñárritu, A. G. USA
There will be blood (2007) Anderson P. T. USA
The Conversation (1974) Coppola, F. F. USA
The Dead (1987) Huston, J. USA
The Godfather 2 (1974) Coppola, F. F. USA
The Good the Bad and the Ugly (1966) Leone, S. USA
The Imposter (2012) Layton, B. UK
The Misfits (1961) Huston, J. USA
The Rider (2017) Zhao, C. USA
The Road (2009) Hillcoat, J. USA

INDEX

Note: Page numbers in *italics* indicate figures

For Product Safety Concerns and Information please contact our EU representative GPSR@taylorandfrancis.com
Taylor & Francis Verlag GmbH, Kaufingerstraße 24, 80331 München, Germany

www.ingramcontent.com/pod-product-compliance
Ingram Content Group UK Ltd.
Pitfield, Milton Keynes, MK11 3LW, UK
UKHW022021180926
475701UK00005B/960

* 9 7 8 1 0 3 2 0 7 2 6 6 1 *